SpringerBriefs in Statistics

For further volumes:
http://www.springer.com/series/8921

Ton J. Cleophas · Aeilko H. Zwinderman

Machine Learning in Medicine—Cookbook Two

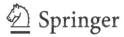 Springer

Ton J. Cleophas
Department Medicine
Albert Schweitzer Hospital
Sliedrecht
The Netherlands

Aeilko H. Zwinderman
Department Biostatistics
  and Epidemiology
Academic Medical Center
Leiden
The Netherlands

Additional material to this book can be downloaded from http://extras.springer.com.

ISSN 2191-544X   ISSN 2191-5458   (electronic)
ISBN 978-3-319-07412-2   ISBN 978-3-319-07413-9   (eBook)
DOI 10.1007/978-3-319-07413-9
Springer Cham Heidelberg New York Dordrecht London

Library of Congress Control Number: 2013957369

Printed on acid-free paper

Springer is part of Springer Science+Business Media (www.springer.com)

Preface

The amount of data stored in the world's medical databases doubles every 20 months, and adequate health and health care will soon be impossible without proper data supervision from modern machine learning methodologies like cluster models, neural networks, and other data mining methodologies. In the past three years we completed three textbooks entitled "Machine Learning in Medicine Part One, Two, and Three" (ed. by Springer Heidelberg Germany, 2012–2013).

It came to our attention that physicians and students often lacked time to read the entire books, and requested a small book, without background information and theoretical discussions, and highlighting technical details. For this reason we produced a 100-page cookbook, entitled "Machine Learning in Medicine—Cookbook One," with data examples available at extras.springer.com for readers to perform their own analyses, and with reference to the above textbooks for those wishing background information. Already at the completion of this cookbook we came to realize that many essential machine learning methods were not covered. The current volume entitled "Machine Learning in Medicine—Cookbook Two" is complementary to the first. It is also intended for providing a more balanced view of the field, and as a must-read not only for physicians and students, but also for any one involved in the process and progress of health and health care.

Similar to the first cookbook, the current work will describe in a nonmathematical way the stepwise analyses of 20 machine learning methods, that are, likewise, based on three major machine learning methodologies:

Cluster Methodologies (Chaps. 1–3),
Linear Methodologies (Chaps. 4–11),
Rules Methodologies (Chaps. 12–20).

In extras.springer.com the data files of the examples are given (both real and hypothesized data), as well as eXtended Markup Language (XML), SPS (Syntax), and ZIP (compressed) files for outcome predictions in future patients. In addition to condensed versions of the methods, fully described in the three textbooks, a first introduction is given to SPSS Modeler (SPSS' data mining workbench) in the Chaps. 15, 18, and 19, while improved statistical methods like various automated analyses and simulation models are in Chaps. 1, 5, 7 and 8.

The current 100-page book entitled "Machine Learning in Medicine—Cookbook Two," and its complementary "Cookbook One" are written as training companions for the 40 most important machine learning methods relevant to medicine. We should emphasize that all of the methods described have been successfully applied in the authors' own research.

Lyon, France, April 2014   Ton J. Cleophas
                                                                Aeilko H. Zwinderman

Contents

Part I
Cluster Models

Chapter 1
Nearest Neighbors for Classifying New Medicines (2 New and 25 Old Opioids)

1.1 General Purpose

Nearest neighbor methodology has a long history, and has, initially, been used for data imputation in demographic data files. This chapter is to assess whether it can also been used for classifying new medicines.

1.2 Specific Scientific Question

For most diseases a whole class of drugs rather than a single compound is available. Nearest neighbor methods can be used for identifying the place of a new drug within its class.

1.3 Example

Two newly developed opioid compounds are assessed for their similarities with the standard opioids in order to determine their potential places in therapeutic regimens. Underneath are the characteristics of 25 standard opioids and two newly developed opioid compounds.

T. J. Cleophas and A. H. Zwinderman, *Machine Learning in Medicine—Cookbook Two*, SpringerBriefs in Statistics, DOI: 10.1007/978-3-319-07413-9_1, © The Author(s) 2014

Drugname	Analgesia score	Antitussive score	Constipation score	Respiratory score	Abuse score	Eliminate time	Duration time
Buprenorphine	7.00	4.00	5.00	7.00	4.00	5.00	9.00
Butorphanol	7.00	3.00	4.00	7.00	4.00	2.70	4.00
Codeine	5.00	6.00	6.00	5.00	4.00	2.90	7.00
Heroine	8.00	6.00	8.00	8.00	10.00	9.00	15.00
Hydromorphone	8.00	6.00	6.00	8.00	8.00	2.60	5.00
Levorphanol	8.00	6.00	6.00	8.00	8.00	11.00	20.00
Mepriridine	7.00	2.00	4.00	8.00	6.00	3.20	14.00
Methadone	9.00	6.00	6.00	8.00	6.00	25.00	5.00
Morphine	8.00	6.00	8.00	8.00	8.00	3.10	5.00
Nalbuphine	7.00	2.00	4.00	7.00	4.00	5.10	4.50
Oxycodone	6.00	6.00	6.00	6.00	8.00	5.00	4.00
Oxymorphine	8.00	5.00	6.00	8.00	8.00	5.20	3.50
Pentazocine	7.00	2.00	4.00	7.00	5.00	2.90	3.00
Propoxyphene	5.00	2.00	4.00	5.00	5.00	3.30	2.00
Nalorphine	2.00	3.00	6.00	8.00	1.00	1.40	3.20
Levallorphan	3.00	2.00	5.00	4.00	1.00	11.00	5.00
Cyclazocine	2.00	3.00	6.00	3.00	2.00	1.60	2.80
Naloxone	1.00	2.00	5.00	8.00	1.00	1.20	3.00
Naltrexone	1.00	3.00	5.00	8.00	0.00	9.70	14.00
Alfentanil	7.00	6.00	7.00	4.00	6.00	1.60	0.50
Alphaprodine	6.00	5.00	6.00	3.00	5.00	2.20	2.00
Fentanyl	6.00	5.00	7.00	5.00	4.00	3.70	0.50

(continued)

(continued)

Drugname	Analgesia score	Antitussive score	Constipation score	Respiratory score	Abuse score	Eliminate time	Duration time
Meptazinol	4.00	3.00	5.00	5.00	3.00	1.60	2.00
Norpropoxyphene	8.00	6.00	8.00	5.00	7.00	6.00	4.00
Sufentanil	7.00	6.00	8.00	6.00	8.00	2.60	5.00
Newdrug1	5.00	5.00	4.00	3.00	6.00	5.00	12.00
Newdrug2	8.00	6.00	3.00	4.00	5.00	7.00	16.00

Var = variable
Var 1 analgesia score (0–10)
Var 2 antitussive score (0–10)
Var 3 constipation score (0–10)
Var 4 respiratory depression score (1–10)
Var 5 abuse liability score (1–10)
Var 6 elimination time ($t_{1/2}$ in hours)
Var 7 duration time analgesia (hours)

The data file is entitled "Chap1nearestneighbor" and is in extras.springer.com.
SPSS statistical software is used for data analysis. Start by opening the data file.
The drug names included, eight variables are in the file. A ninth variable entitled
"partition" must be added with the value 1 for the opioids 1–25 and 0 for the two
new compounds (cases 26 and 27).

Then command:

Analyze...Classify...Nearest Neighbor Analysis...enter the variable "drugs-
name" in Target...enter the variables "analgesia" to "duration of analgesia" in
Features...click Partitions...click Use variable to assign cases...enter the variable
"Partition"....click OK.

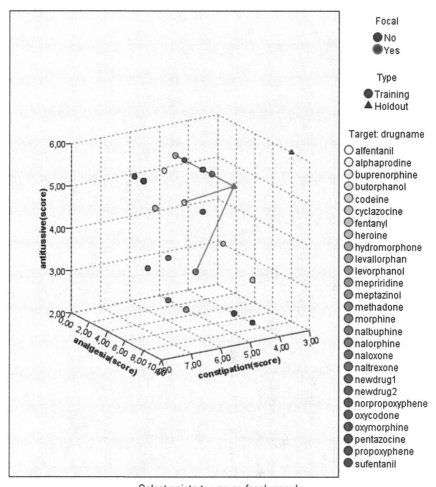

Select points to use as focal records

This chart is a lower-dimensional projection of the predictor space, which contains a total of 7
predictors.

The above figure shows as an example the place of the two new compounds (the small triangles) as compared with those of the standard opioids. Lines connect them to their three nearest neighbors. In SPSS' original output sheets the graph can by double-clicking be placed in the "model viewer", and, then, (after again clicking on it) be interactively rotated in order to improve the view of the distances. SPSS uses three nearest neighbors by default, but you can change this number if you like. The names of the compounds are given in alphabetical order. Only three of seven variables

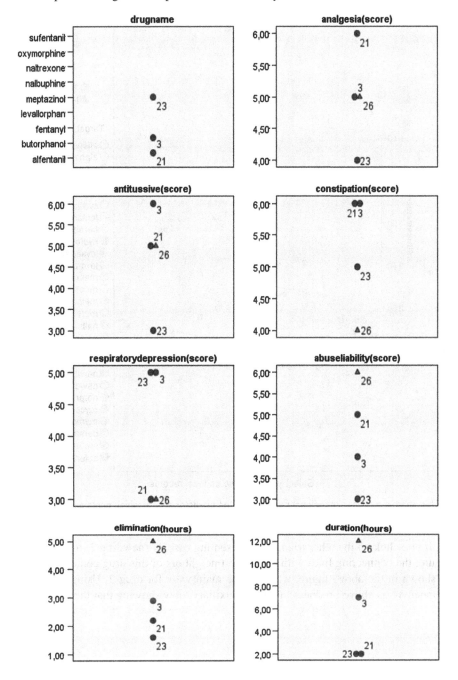

are given in the initial figure, but if you click on one of the small triangles in this figure, an auxiliary view comes up right from the main view. Here are all the details of the analysis. The upper left graph of it shows that the opioids 21, 3, and 23 have the best average nearest neighbor records for case 26 (new drug 1). The seven figures alongside and underneath this figure give the distances between these three and case 26 for each of the seven features (otherwise called predictor variables).

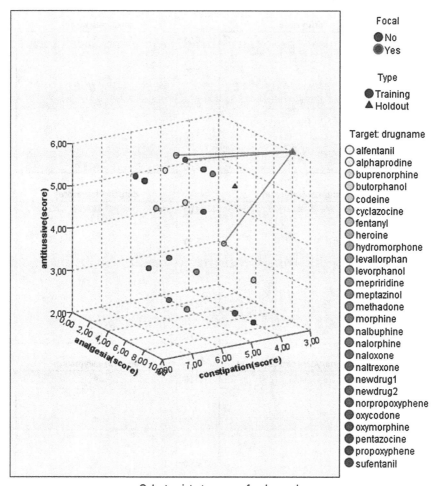

Select points to use as focal records

This chart is a lower-dimensional projection of the predictor space, which contains a total of 7 predictors.

If you click on the other triangle (representing case 27 (newdrug 2) in the initial figure, the connecting lines with the nearest neighbors of this drug comes up. This is shown in the above figure, which is the main view for drug 2. Using the same manoeuvre as above produces again the auxiliary view showing that the opioids 3,

1, and 11 have the best average nearest neighbor records for case 27 (new drug 2). The seven figures alongside and underneath this figure give again the distances between these three and case 27 for each of the seven features (otherwise called predictor variables). The auxiliary view is shown underneath.

Peers Chart
Focal Records and Nearest Neighbors

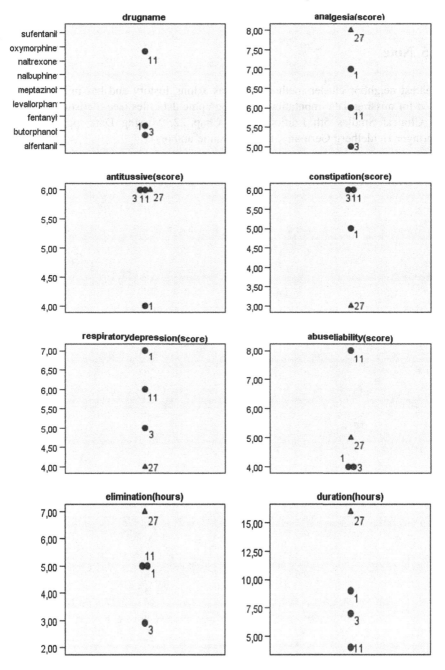

1.4 Conclusion

Nearest neighbor methodology enables to readily identify the places of new drugs within their classes of drugs. For example, newly developed opioid compounds can be compared with standard opioids in order to determine their potential places in therapeutic regimens.

1.5 Note

Nearest neighbor cluster methodology has a long history and has initially been used for missing data imputation in demographic data files (see Statistics Applied to Clinical Studies 5th Edition, 2012, Chap. 22, Missing Data, pp 253–266, Springer Heidelberg Germany, from the same authors).

Chapter 2
Predicting High-Risk-Bin Memberships (1,445 Families)

2.1 General Purpose

Optimal bins describe continuous predictor variables in the form of best fit categories for making predictions, e.g., about families at high risk of bank loan defaults. In addition, it can be used for, e.g., predicting health risk cut-offs about individual future families, based on their characteristics.

2.2 Specific Scientific Question

Can optimal binning also be applied for other medical purposes, e.g., for finding high risk cut-offs for overweight children in particular families?

2.3 Example

A data file of 1,445 families was assessed for learning the best fit cut-off values of unhealthy lifestyle estimators to maximize the difference between low and high risk of overweight children. These cut-off values were, subsequently, used to determine the risk profiles (the characteristics) in individual future families.

Var 1	Var 2	Var 3	Var 4	Var 5
0	11	1	8	0
0	7	1	9	0
1	25	7	0	1
0	11	4	5	0
1	5	1	8	1
0	10	2	8	0
0	11	1	6	0
0	7	1	8	0
0	7	0	9	0
0	15	3	0	0

Var = variable
Var 1fruitvegetables (times per week)
Var 2 unhealthysnacks (times per week)
Var 3 fastfoodmeal (times per week)
Var 4 physicalactivities (times per week)
Var 5 overweightchildren (0 = no, 1 = yes)

Only the first 10 families of the original learning data file are given, the entire data file is entitled "chap2optimalbinning" and is in extras.springer.com.

2.4 Optimal Binning

SPSS 19.0 is used for analysis. Start by opening the data file.
Command:
Transform...Optimal Binning...Variables into Bins: enter fruitvegetables, un-healthysnacks, fastfoodmeal, physicalactivities...Optimize Bins with Respect to: enter "overweightchildren"...click Output...Display: mark Endpoints...mark Descriptive statistics...mark Model Entropy...click Save: mark Create variables that contain binned data...Save Binning Rules in a Syntax file: click Browse...open appropriate folder...File name: enter, e.g., "exportoptimalbinning"...click Save...click OK.

fruitvegetables/wk

Bin	End point		Number of cases by level of overweight children		
	Lower	Upper	No	Yes	Total
1	a	14	802	340	1,142
2	14	a	274	29	303
Total			1076	369	1,445

unhealthysnacks/wk

Bin	End point		Number of cases by level of overweight children		
	Lower	Upper	No	Yes	Total
1	a	12	830	143	973
2	12	19	188	126	314
3	19	a	58	100	158
Total			1,076	369	1,445

fastfoodmeal/wk

Bin	End point		Number of cases by level of overweight children		
	Lower	Upper	No	Yes	Total
1	a	2	896	229	1,125
2	2	a	180	140	320
Total			1,076	369	1,445

physicalactivities/wk

Bin	End point		Number of cases by level of overweight children		
	Lower	Upper	No	Yes	Total
1	a	8	469	221	690
2	8	a	607	148	755
Total			1,076	369	1,445

Each bin is computed as lower <= physical activities/wk < Upper
[a] Unbounded

In the output sheets the above table is given. It shows the high risk cut-offs for overweight children of the four predicting factors. E.g., in 1,142 families scoring under 14 units of (1) fruit/vegetable per week, are put into bin 1 and 303 scoring over 14 units per week, are put into bin 2. The proportion of overweight children in bin 1 is much larger than it is in bin 2: $340/1142 = 0.298$ (30 %) and $29/303 = 0.096$ (10 %). Similarly high risk cut-offs are found for (2) unhealthy snacks less than 12, 12–19, and over 19 per week, (3) fastfood meals less than 2, and over 2 per week, (4) physical activities less than 8 and over 8 per week. These cut-offs will be used as meaningful recommendation limits to eleven future families.

Fruit	Snacks	Fastfood	Physical
13	11	4	5
2	5	3	9
12	23	9	0
17	9	6	5
2	3	3	3
10	8	4	3
15	9	3	6
9	5	3	8

(continued)

(continued)

Fruit	Snacks	Fastfood	Physical
2	5	2	7
9	13	5	0
28	3	3	9

Var 1fruitvegetables (times per week)
Var 2 unhealthysnacks (times per week)
Var 3 fastfoodmeal (times per week)
Var 4 physicalactivities (times per week)

The saved syntax file entitled "exportoptimalbinning.sps" will now be used to compute the predicted bins of some future families. Enter the above values in a new data file, entitled, e.g., "chap2optimalbinning2", and save in the appropriate folder in your computer. Then open up the data file "exportoptimalbinning.sps" …subsequently click File…click Open…click Data…Find the data file entitled "optimalbinning2"…click Open…click "exportoptimalbinning.sps" from the file palette at the bottom of the screen…click Run…click All.

When returning to the Data View of "chap2optimalbinning2", we will find the underneath overview of all of the bins selected for our eleven future families.

Fruit	Snacks	Fastfood	Physical	Fruit	Snacks	Fastfood	Physical
				_bin	_bin	_bin	_bin
13	11	4	5	1	1	2	1
2	5	3	9	1	1	2	2
12	23	9	0	1	3	2	1
17	9	6	5	2	1	2	1
2	3	3	3	1	1	2	1
10	8	4	3	1	1	2	1
15	9	3	6	2	1	2	1
9	5	3	8	1	1	2	2
2	5	2	7	1	1	2	1
9	13	5	0	1	2	2	1
28	3	3	9	2	1	2	2

This overview is relevant, since families in high risk bins would particularly qualify for counseling.

2.5 Conclusion

Optimal bins describe continuous predictor variables in the form of best fit categories for making predictions, and SPSS statistical software can be used to generate a syntax file, called SPS file, for predicting risk cut-offs in future families. In
this way families highly at risk for overweight can be readily identified. The nodes
of decision trees can be used for similar purposes (Machine learning in medicine
Cookbook One, Chap. 16, Decision trees for decision analysis, pp 97–104,
Springer Heidelberg Germany, 2,014), but it has subgroups of cases, rather than
multiple bins for a single case.

2.6 Note

More background, theoretical and mathematical information of optimal binning is
given in Machine Learning in Medicine Part Three, Chap. 5, Optimal binning,
pp 37–48, Springer Heidelberg Germany 2013, and Machine learning in medicine
Cookbook One, Optimal binning, Chap. 19, pp 101–106, Springer Heidelberg
Germany, 2014, both from the same authors.

Chapter 3
Predicting Outlier Memberships
(2,000 Patients)

3.1 General Purpose

With large data files outlier recognition requires a more sophisticated approach than the traditional data plots and regression lines. This chapter is to examine whether BIRCH (balanced iterative reducing and clustering using hierarchies) clustering is able to predict outliers in future patients from a known population.

3.2 Specific Scientific Question

Is the XML (eXtended Markup Language) file from a 2,000 patient sample capable of making predictions about cluster memberships and outlierships in future patients from the target population.

3.3 Example

In a 2,000 patient study of hospital admissions 576 possibly iatrogenic admissions were identified. Based on age and numbers of co-medications a two step BIRCH cluster analysis will be performed. SPSS version 19 and up can be used for the purpose. Only the first 10 patients' data are shown underneath. The entire data file is in extras.springer.com, and is entitled "chap3outlierdetection".

T. J. Cleophas and A. H. Zwinderman, *Machine Learning in Medicine—Cookbook Two*, SpringerBriefs in Statistics, DOI: 10.1007/978-3-319-07413-9_3, © The Author(s) 2014

Age	Gender	Admis	Duration	Mort	Iatro	Comorb	Comed
1939.00	2.00	7.00	0.00	0.00	1.00	2.00	1.00
1939.00	2.00	7.00	2.00	1.00	1.00	2.00	1.00
1943.00	2.00	11.00	1.00	0.00	1.00	0.00	0.00
1921.00	2.00	9.00	17.00	0.00	1.00	3.00	3.00
1944.00	2.00	21.00	30.00	0.00	1.00	3.00	3.00
1977.00	2.00	4.00	1.00	0.00	1.00	1.00	1.00
1930.00	1.00	20.00	7.00	0.00	1.00	2.00	2.00
1932.00	1.00	3.00	2.00	0.00	1.00	4.00	4.00
1927.00	1.00	9.00	13.00	1.00	1.00	1.00	2.00
1920.00	2.00	23.00	8.00	0.00	1.00	3.00	3.00

admis = admission indication code
duration = days of admission
mort = mortality
iatro = iatrogenic admission
comorb = number of comorbidities
comed = number of comedications

Start by opening the file. Then command:

click Transform....click Random Number Generators....click Set Starting Point....click Fixed Value (2,000,000)....click OK....click Analyze.... Classify....Two Step Cluster Analysis ....Continuous Variables: enter age and co-medications....Distance Measure: mark Euclidean....Clustering Criterion: mark Schwarz's Bayesian Criterion....click Options: mark Use noise handling ....percentage: enter 25....Assumed Standardized: enter age and co-medications ....click Continue....mark Pivot tables....mark Charts and tables in Model Viewer....Working Data File: mark Create Cluster membership variable....XML Files: mark Export final model....click Browse....select the appropriate folder in your computer....File Name: enter, e.g., "exportanomalydetection"....click Save....click Continue....click OK.

In the output sheets the underneath distribution of clusters is given.

Cluster distribution			
	N	% of combined	% of total
Cluster 1	181	31.4	9.1
2	152	26.4	7.6
3	69	12.0	3.5
Outlier (−1)	174	30.2	8.7
Combined	576	100.0	28.8
Excluded cases	1,424		71.2
Total	2,000		100.0

Additional details are given in Machine learning in medicine Part Two, Chap. 10, Anomaly detection, pp 93–103, Springer Heidelberg, Germany, 2013. The large outlier category consisted mainly of patients of all ages and extremely many co-medications. When returning to the Data View screen, we will observe that SPSS has created a novel variable entitled "TSC_5980" containing the patients' cluster memberships. The patients given the value −1 are the outliers.

With Scoring Wizard and the exported XML (eXtended Markup Language) file entitled "exportanomalydetection" we can now try and predict from age and number of co-medications of future patients the best fit cluster membership according to the computed XML model.

Age	Comed
1954.00	1.00
1938.00	7.00
1929.00	8.00
1967.00	1.00
1945.00	2.00
1936.00	3.00
1928.00	4.00

comed = number of co-medications

Enter the above data in a novel data file and command:

Utilities....click Scoring Wizard....click Browse....Open the appropriate folder with the XML file entitled "exportanomalydetection"....click on the latter and click Select....in Scoring Wizard double-click Next....mark Predicted Value ....click Finish.

Age	Comed	Predicted value
1954.00	1.00	3.00
1938.00	7.00	−1.00
1929.00	8.00	−1.00
1967.00	1.00	3.00
1945.00	2.00	−1.00
1936.00	3.00	1.00
1928.00	4.00	−1.00

Predicted Value = predicted cluster membership

In the above novel data file SPSS has provided the new variable as requested. One patient is in cluster 1, two are in cluster 3, and 4 patients are in the outlier cluster.

3.4 Conclusion

An XML (eXtended Markup Language) file from a 2,000 patient sample is capable of making predictions about cluster memberships and outlierships in future patients from the same target population.

3.5 Note

More background theoretical and mathematical information of outlier detection is available in Machine learning in medicine Part Two, Chap.10, Anomaly detection, pp 93–103, Springer Heidelberg Germany, 2013, from the same authors.

Part II
Linear Models

Chapter 4
Polynomial Regression for Outcome Categories (55 Patients)

4.1 General Purpose

To assess whether polynomial regression can be trained to make predictions about (1) patients being in a category and (2) the probability of it.

4.2 Specific Scientific Question

Patients from different hospital departments and ages are assessed for falling out of bed (0 = no, 1 = yes without injury, 2 = yes with injury). The falloutofbed categories are the outcome, the department and ages are the predictors. Can a data file of such patients be trained to make predictions in future patients about their best fit category and probability of being in it.

Department	Falloutofbed	Age (years)
0.00	1	56.00
0.00	1	58.00
0.00	1	87.00
0.00	1	64.00
0.00	1	65.00
0.00	1	53.00
0.00	1	87.00
0.00	1	77.00
0.00	1	78.00
0.00	1	89.00

Only the first 10 patients are given, the entire data file is entitled "chap4categoriesasoutcome" and is in extras.springer.com.

T. J. Cleophas and A. H. Zwinderman, *Machine Learning in Medicine—Cookbook Two*, SpringerBriefs in Statistics, DOI: 10.1007/978-3-319-07413-9_4, © The Author(s) 2014

4.3 The Computer Teaches Itself to Make Predictions

SPSS versions 18 and later can be used. SPSS will produce an XML (eXtended Markup Language) file of the prediction model from the above data. We will start by opening the above data file.

Command: click Transform....click Random Number Generators....click Set Starting Point....click Fixed Value (2,000,000)....click OK....click Analyze.... Regression ....Multinomial Logistic Regression....Dependent: falloutofbed....

Factor: department....Covariate: age....click Save....mark: Estimated response probability, Predicted category, Predicted category probability, Actual category probability....click Browse....various folders in your personal computer come up....in "File name" of the appropriate folder enter "exportcategoriesasoutcome" ....click Save....click Continue....click OK.

Parameter estimates								
Fall with/out injury[a]	B	Std. error	Wald	df	Sig.	Exp. (B)	95 % confidence interval for Exp. (B)	
							Lower bound	Upper bound
0 Intercept	5.337	2.298	5.393	1	0.020			
Age	−0.059	0.029	4.013	1	0.045	0.943	0.890	0.999
(Department = 0.00)	−1.139	0.949	1.440	1	0.230	0.320	0.050	2.057
(Department = 1.00)	0[b]	.	.	0	.	.	.	.
1 Intercept	3.493	2.333	2.241	1	0.134			
Age	−0.022	0.029	0.560	1	0.454	0.978	0.924	1.036
(Department = 0.00)	−1.945	0.894	4.735	1	0.030	0.143	0.025	0.824
(Department = 1.00)	0[b]	.	.	0	.	.	.	.

[a] The reference catagory is: 2
[b] This parameter is set to zero because it is redundant

The above table is in the output. The independent predictors of falloutofbed are given. Per year of age there are 0.943 less "no falloutofbeds" versus "falloutofbeds with injury". The department 0.00 has 0.143 less falloutofbeds with versus without injury. The respective p-values are 0.045 and 0.030. When returning to the main data view, we will observe that SPSS has provided 6 novel variables for each patient.

1. EST1_1 estimated response probability (probability of the category 0 for each patient)
2. EST2_1 idem for category 1

3. EST3_1 idem for category 2
4. PRE_1 predicted category (category with highest probability score)
5. PCP_1 predicted category probability (the highest probability score predicted by model)
6. ACP_1 actual category probability (the highest probability computed from data).

With the Scoring Wizard and the exported XML file entitled "exportcategoriesasoutcome" we can now try and predict from the department and age of future patients (1) the most probable category they are in, and (2) the very probability of it. The department and age of 12 novel patients are as follow.
Enter the above data in a novel data file and command:

Department	Age
0.00	73.00
0.00	38.00
1.00	89.00
0.00	75.00
0.00	84.00
0.00	74.00
1.00	90.00
1.00	72.00
1.00	62.00
1.00	34.00
1.00	85.00
1.00	43.00

Utilities....click Scoring Wizard....click Browse....Open the appropriate folder with the XML file entitled "exportcategoriesasoutcome"....click on the latter and click Select....in Scoring Wizard double-click Next....mark Predicted category and Probability of it....click Finish.

Department	Age	Probability of being in predicted category	Predicted category
0.00	73.00	0.48	1.00
0.00	38.00	0.48	1.00
1.00	89.00	0.36	2.00
0.00	75.00	0.47	1.00
0.00	84.00	0.48	2.00
0.00	74.00	0.48	1.00
1.00	90.00	0.37	2.00
1.00	72.00	0.55	0.00
1.00	62.00	0.65	0.00
1.00	34.00	0.84	0.00

(continued)

(continued)

Department	Age	Probability of being in predicted category	Predicted category
1.00	85.00	0.39	0.00
1.00	43.00	0.79	0.00

0 = no falloutofbed
1 = falloutofbed without injury
2 = falloutofbed with injury

In the data file SPSS has provided two novel variables as requested. The first patient from department 0.00 and 73 years of age has a 48 % chance of being in the "falloutofbed without injury". His/her chance of being in the other two categories is smaller than 48 %.

4.4 Conclusion

Multinomial or polynomial logistic regression can be readily trained to make predictions in future patients about their best fit category and the probability of being in it.

4.5 Note

More background theoretical and mathematical information of analyses using categories as outcome is available in Machine Learning in Medicine Part Two, Chap. 10, Anomaly detection, pp 93–103, Springer Heidelberg Germany, 2013.

Chapter 5
Automatic Nonparametric Tests for Predictor Categories (60 and 30 Patients)

5.1 General Purpose

Categories unlike continuous data need not have stepping functions. In order to apply regression analysis for their analysis we need to recode them into multiple binary (dummy) variables. Particularly, if Gaussian distributions in the outcome are uncertain, automatic non-parametric testing is an adequate and very convenient modern alternative.

5.2 Specific Scientific Questions

1. Does race have an effect on physical strength (the variable race has a categorical rather than linear pattern).
2. Are the hours of sleep / levels of side effects different in categories treated with different sleeping pills.

5.3 Example 1

The effects on physical strength (scores 0–100) assessed in 60 subjects of different races hispanics (1), blacks (2), asians (3), and whites (4), and ages (years), are in the left three columns of the data file entitled "chap5categoriesaspredictor".

T. J. Cleophas and A. H. Zwinderman, *Machine Learning in Medicine—Cookbook Two*, SpringerBriefs in Statistics, DOI: 10.1007/978-3-319-07413-9_5, © The Author(s) 2014

Patient number	Physical strength	Race	Age
1	70.00	1.00	35.00
2	77.00	1.00	55.00
3	66.00	1.00	70.00
4	59.00	1.00	55.00
5	71.00	1.00	45.00
6	72.00	1.00	47.00
7	45.00	1.00	75.00
8	85.00	1.00	83.00
9	70.00	1.00	35.00
10	77.00	1.00	49.00

Only the first 10 patients are displayed above. The entire data file in www.springer.com. For the analysis we will use multiple linear regression.

Command:

Analyze....Regression....Linear....Dependent: physical strength score.... Independent: race, age, ...OK.

Coefficients[a]

Model	Unstandardized coefficients		Standardized coefficients	t	Sig.
	B	Std. error	Beta		
1 (Constant)	92.920	7.640		12.162	0.000
Race	−0.330	1.505	−0.027	−0.219	0.827
Age	−0.356	0.116	−0.383	−3.071	0.003

[a] *Dependent variable* Strengthscore

The above table shows that age is a significant predictor but race is not. However, the analysis is not adequate, because the variable race is analyzed as a stepwise function from 1 to 4, and the linear regression model assumes that the outcome variable will rise (or fall) linearly, but, in the data given, this needs not be necessarily so. It may, therefore, be more safe to recode the stepping variable into the form of a categorical variable. The underneath data overview shows in the right 4 columns how it is manually done.

Patient number	Physical strength	Race	Age	Race 1 hispanics	Race 2 blacks	Race 3 asians	Race 4 whites
1	70.00	1.00	35.00	1.00	0.00	0.00	0.00
2	77.00	1.00	55.00	1.00	0.00	0.00	0.00
3	66.00	1.00	70.00	1.00	0.00	0.00	0.00
4	59.00	1.00	55.00	1.00	0.00	0.00	0.00

(continued)

(continued)

Patient number	Physical strength	Race	Age	Race 1 hispanics	Race 2 blacks	Race 3 asians	Race 4 whites
5	71.00	1.00	45.00	1.00	0.00	0.00	0.00
6	72.00	1.00	47.00	1.00	0.00	0.00	0.00
7	45.00	1.00	75.00	1.00	0.00	0.00	0.00
8	85.00	1.00	83.00	1.00	0.00	0.00	0.00
9	70.00	1.00	35.00	1.00	0.00	0.00	0.00
10	77.00	1.00	49.00	1.00	0.00	0.00	0.00

We. subsequently, use again linear regression, but now for categorical analysis of race.

Command:

click Transform....click Random Number Generators....click Set Starting Point....
click Fixed Value (2000000)....click OK....click Analyze....Regression
....Linear
....Dependent: physical strength score....Independent: race 1, race 3, race 4, age....
click Save....mark Unstandardized....in Export model information to XML (eXtended Markup Language) file: type "exportcategoriesaspredictor"....click Browse....File name: enter "exportcategoriesaspredictor"....click Continue....click OK.

Coefficients[a]

Model	Unstandardized coefficients		Standardized coefficients	t	Sig.
	B	Std. error	Beta		
1 (Constant)	97.270	4.509		21.572	0.000
Age	−0.200	0.081	−0.215	−2.457	0.017
Race1	−17.483	3.211	−0.560	−5.445	0.000
Race3	−25.670	3.224	−0.823	−7.962	0.000
Race4	−8.811	3.198	−0.282	−2.755	0.008

[a] *Dependent variable* Strengthscore

The above table is in the output. It shows that race 1, 3, 4 are significant predictors of physical strength compared to race 2. The results can be interpreted as follows.

The underneath regression equation is used:

$$y = a + b_1 x_1 + b_2 x_2 + b_3 x_3 + b_4 x_4$$

$a =$ intercept
$b_1 =$ regression coefficient for age
$b_2 =$ hispanics

$b_3 =$ asians
$b_4 =$ white

If an individual is black (race 2), then x_2, x_3, and x_4 will turn into 0, and the regression equation becomes

	$y = a + b_1 x_1$
If hispanic,	$y = a + b_1 x_1 + b_2 x_2$
If asian,	$y = a + b_1 x_1 + b_3 x_3$
If white,	$y = a + b_1 x_1 + b_4 x_4.$

So, e.g., the best predicted physical strength score of a white male of 25 years of age would equal

$y = 97.270 + 0.20 * 25 - 8.811*1 = 93.459,$

($* =$ sign of multiplication).

Obviously, all of the races are negative predictors of physical strength, but the blacks scored highest and the asians lowest. All of these results are adjusted for age.

If we return to the data file page, we will observe that SPSS has added a new variable entitled "PRE_1". It represents the individual strengthscores as predicted by the recoded linear model. They are pretty similar to the measured values.

We can now with the help of the Scoring Wizard and the exported XML (eXtended Markup Language) file entitled "exportcategoriesaspredictor" try and predict strength scores of future patients with known race and age.

Race	Age
1.00	40.00
2.00	70.00
3.00	54.00
4.00	45.00
1.00	36.00
2.00	46.00
3.00	50.00
4.00	36.00

First, recode the stepping variable race into 4 categorical variables.

Race	Age	Race1	Race3	Race4
1.00	40.00	1.00	0.00	0.00
2.00	70.00	0.00	0.00	0.00
3.00	54.00	0.00	1.00	0.00
4.00	45.00	0.00	0.00	1.00
1.00	36.00	1.00	0.00	0.00
2.00	46.00	0.00	0.00	0.00
3.00	50.00	0.00	1.00	0.00
4.00	36.00	0.00	0.00	1.00

Then command:

click Utilities....click Scoring Wizard....click Browse....click Select....Folder: enter the exportcategoriesaspredictor.xml file....click Select....in Scoring Wizard click Next....click Finish.

Race	Age	Race1	Race3	Race4	Predicted strength score
1.00	40.00	1.00	0.00	0.00	71.81
2.00	70.00	0.00	0.00	0.00	83.30
3.00	54.00	0.00	1.00	0.00	60.83
4.00	45.00	0.00	0.00	1.00	79.48
1.00	36.00	1.00	0.00	0.00	72.60
2.00	46.00	0.00	0.00	0.00	88.09
3.00	50.00	0.00	1.00	0.00	61.62
4.00	36.00	0.00	0.00	1.00	81.28

The above data file now gives predicted strength scores of the 8 future patients as computed with help of the XML file.

Also with a binary outcome variable categorical analysis of covariates is possible. Using logistic regression in SPSS is convenient for the purpose, we need not *manually* transform the quantitative estimator into a categorical one. For the analysis we have to apply the usual commands.

Command: Analyze ....Regression....Binary logistic....Dependent variable.... Independent variables....then, open dialog box labeled Categorical Variables.... select the categorical variable and transfer it to the box Categorical Variables....then click Continue....OK.

5.4 Example 2

Particularly, if Gaussian distributions in the outcome are uncertain, automatic non-parametric testing is an adequate and very convenient modern alternative. Three parallel-groups were treated with different sleeping pills. Both hours of sleep and side effect score were assessed.

Group	Efficacy	Gender	Comorbidity	Side effect score
0	6.00	0.00	1.00	45.00
0	7.10	0.00	1.00	35.00
0	8.10	0.00	0.00	34.00
0	7.50	0.00	0.00	29.00
0	6.40	0.00	1.00	480.00
0	7.90	1.00	1.00	23.00
0	6.80	1.00	1.00	56.00
0	6.60	1.00	.00	54.00
0	7.30	1.00	0.00	33.00
0	5.60	0.00	0.00	75.00

Only the first ten patients are shown. The entire data file is in extras.springer.com and is entitled "chap5categoriesaspredictor2". Automatic non-parametric tests is available in SPSS 18 and up. Start by opening the above data file.

Command:

Analyze....Nonparametric Tests....Independent Samples....click Objective.... mark Automatically compare distributions across groups....click Fields....in Test fields: enter "hours of sleep" and "side effect score"....in Groups: enter "group"....click Settings....Choose Tests....mark "Automatically choose the tests based on the data"....click Run.

In the interactive output sheets the underneath table is given. Both the distribution of hours of sleep and side effect score are significantly different across the three categories of treatment. The traditional assessment of these data would have been a multivariate analysis of variance (MANOVA) with treatment-category as predictor and both hours of sleep and side effect score as outcome. However, normal distributions are uncertain in this example, and the correlation between the two outcome measures may not be zero, reducing the sensitivity of MANOVA. A nice thing about the automatic nonparametric tests is that, like discriminant analysis (Machine Learning in Medicine Part One, Chap. 17, Discriminant analysis for supervised data, pp 215–224, Springer Heidelberg Germany, 2013), they assume orthogonality of the two outcomes, which means that the correlation level between the two does not have to be taken into account. By double-clicking the table you will obtain an interactive set of views of various details of the analysis, entitled the Model Viewer.

Hypothesis Test Summary

	Null Hypothesis	Test	Sig.	Decision
1	The distribution of hours of sleep is the same across categories of group.	Independent-Samples Kruskal-Wallis Test	,001	Reject the null hypothesis.
2	The distribution of side effect score is the same across categories of group.	Independent-Samples Kruskal-Wallis Test	,036	Reject the null hypothesis.

Asymptotic significances are displayed. The significance level is ,05.

One view provides the box and whiskers graphs (medians, quartiles, and ranges) of hours of sleep of the three treatment groups. Group 0 seems to perform better than the other two, but we don't know where the significant differences are.

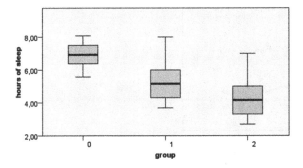

Also the box and whiskers graph of side effect scores is given. Some groups again seem to perform better than the other. However, we cannot see whether 0 versus 1, 1 versus 2, and/or 0 versus 2 are significantly different.

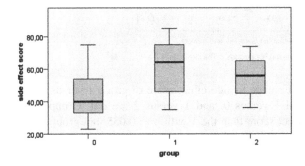

In the view space at the bottom of the auxiliary view (right half of the Model Viewer) several additional options are given. When clicking Pairwise Comparisons, a distance network is displayed with yellow lines corresponding to statistically significant differences, and black ones to insignificant ones. Obviously, the differences in hours of sleep of group 1 versus 0 and group 2 versus 0 are statistically significant, and 1 versus 2 is not. Group 0 had significantly more hours of sleep than the other two groups with p = 0.044 and 0.0001.

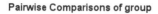

Pairwise Comparisons of group

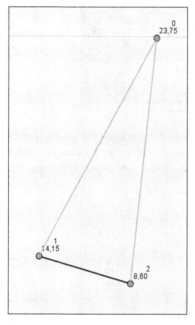

Each node shows the sample average rank of group.

Sample1-Sample2	Test Statistic	Std. Error	Std. Test Statistic	Sig.	Adj.Sig.
2- 1	5,550	3,936	1,410	,158	,475
2- 0	15,150	3,936	3,849	,000	,000
1- 0	9,600	3,936	2,439	,015	,044

Each row tests the null hypothesis that the Sample 1 and Sample 2 distributions are the same.
Asymptotic significances (2-sided tests) are displayed. The significance level is ,05.

As shown below, the difference in side effect score of group 1 versus 0 is also statistically significant, and 1 versus 0, and 1 versus 2 are not. Group 0 has a significantly better side effect score than the 1 with p = 0.035, but group 0 versus 2 and 1 versus 2 are not significantly different.

Pairwise Comparisons of group

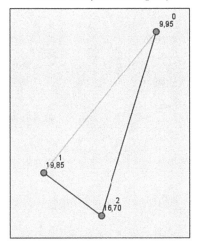

Each node shows the sample average rank of group.

Sample1-Sample2	Test Statistic	Std. Error	Std. Test Statistic	Sig.	Adj.Sig.
0- 2	-6,750	3,931	-1,717	,086	,258
0- 1	-9,900	3,931	-2,518	,012	,035
2- 1	3,150	3,931	,801	,423	1,000

Each row tests the null hypothesis that the Sample 1 and Sample 2
distributions are the same.
Asymptotic significances (2-sided tests) are displayed. The significance level
is ,05.

5.5 Conclusion

Predictor variables with a categorical rather than linear character should be recoded
into categorical variables before analysis in a regression model. An example is
given. Particularly if the Gaussian distributions in the outcome are uncertain,
automatic non-parametric testing is an adequate and very convenient alternative.

5.6 Note

More background theoretical and mathematical information of categories as predictor is given in SPSS for Starters Part Two, Chap. 5, Categorical data, pp 21–24,
and Statistics Applied to Clinical Studies, 5th Edition, Chap. 21, Races as a categorical variable, pp 244-252, both from the same authors and edited by Springer
Heidelberg Germany 2012.

Chapter 6
Random Intercept Models for Both Outcome and Predictor Categories (55 Patients)

6.1 General Purpose

Categories are very common in medical research. Examples include age classes, income classes, education levels, drug dosages, diagnosis groups, disease severities, etc. Statistics has generally difficulty to assess categories, and traditional models require either binary or continuous variables. If in the outcome, categories can be assessed with polynomial regression (see the above Chap. 4), if as predictors, they can be assessed with automatic nonparametric tests (see the above Chap. 5). However, with multiple categories or with categories both in the outcome and as predictors, random intercept models may provide better sensitivity of testing. The latter models assume that for each predictor category or combination of categories x_1, x_2,... slightly different a-values can be computed with a better fit for the outcome category y than a single a-value.

$$y = a + b_1 x_1 + b_2 x_2 + \ldots$$

We should add that, instead of the above linear equation, even better results were obtained with log-linear equations (log = natural logarithm).

$$\log y = a + b_1 x_1 + b_2 x_2 + \ldots$$

6.2 Specific Scientific Question

In a study three hospital departments (no surgery, little surgery, lot of surgery), and three patient age classes (young, middle, old) were the predictors of the risk class of falling out of bed (fall out of bed no, yes but no injury, yes and injury). Are the predictor categories significant determinants of the risk of falling out of bed with or without injury. Does a random intercept provide better statistics.

T. J. Cleophas and A. H. Zwinderman, *Machine Learning in Medicine—Cookbook Two*, SpringerBriefs in Statistics, DOI: 10.1007/978-3-319-07413-9_6, © The Author(s) 2014

6.3 Example

Department	Falloutofbed	Agecat	Patient_id
0	1	1.00	1.00
0	1	1.00	2.00
0	1	2.00	3.00
0	1	1.00	4.00
0	1	1.00	5.00
0	1	0.00	6.00
1	1	2.00	7.00
0	1	2.00	8.00
1	1	2.00	9.00
0	1	0.00	10.00

Variable 1: department = department class (0 = no surgery, 1 = little surgery, 2 = lot of surgery)
Variable 2: falloutofbed = risk of falling out of bed (0 = fall out of bed no, 1 = yes but no injury, 2 = yes and injury)
Variable 3: agecat = patient age classes (young, middle, old)
Variable 4: patient_id = patient identification

Only the first 10 patients of the 55 patient file is shown above. The entire data file is in extras.springer.com and is entitled "Chap6randomintercept.sav". SPSS version 20 and up can be used for analysis. First, we will perform a fixed intercept log-linear analysis.

Command:

click Analyze...click Data Structure...click "patient_id" and drag to Subjects on the Canvas...click Fields and Effects...click Target...Target: select "fall with/out injury"...click Fixed Effects...click "agecat" and "department" and drag to Effect Builder:...mark Include intercept...click Run.

The underneath results show that both the various regression coefficients as well as the overall correlation coefficients between the predictors and the outcome are, generally, statistically significant.

Source	F	df1	df2	Sig.
Corrected Model ▼	9,398	4	10	,002
agecat	6,853	2	10	,013
department	9,839	2	10	,004

Probability distribution:Multinomial
Link function:Cumulative logit

Model Term		Coefficient ▶	Sig.
Threshold for falloutofbed=	0	2,140	,028
	1	7,229	,000
agecat=0		5,236	,005
agecat=1		-0,002	,998
agecat=2		0,000[a]	
department=0		3,660	,008
department=1		4,269	,002
department=2		0,000[a]	

Probability distribution:Multinomial
Link function:Cumulative logit

[a]This coefficient is set to zero because it is redundant.

Subsequently, a random intercept analysis is performed.

Command:

Analyze...click Data Structure...click "patient_id" and drag to Subjects on the Canvas...click Fields and Effects...click Target...Target: select "fall with/out injury"...click Fixed Effects...click "agecat" and "department" and drag to Effect Builder:...mark Include intercept...click Random Effects...click Add Block...– mark Include intercept...Subject combination: select patient_id...click OK...click Model Options...click Save Fields...mark PredictedValue...mark PredictedProbability...click Save...click Run.

The underneath results show the test statistics of the random intercept model. The random intercept model shows better statistics:

p = 0.007 and 0.013	overall for age,
p = 0.001 and 0.004	overall for department,
p = 0.003 and 0.005	regression coefficients for age class 0 versus 2,
p = 0.900 and 0.998	for age class 1 versus 2,
p = 0.004 and 0.008	for department 0 versus 2, and
p = 0.001 and 0.0002	for department 1 versus 2.

Source	F	df1	df2	Sig.
Corrected Model ▼	7,935	4	49	,000
agecat	5,513	2	49	,007
department	7,602	2	49	,001

Probability distribution:Multinomial
Link function:Cumulative logit

Model Term		Coefficient ▶	Sig.
Threshold for falloutofbed=	0	2,082	,015
	1	5,464	,000
agecat=0		3,869	,003
agecat=1		0,096	,900
agecat=2		0,000ᵃ	
department=0		3,228	,004
department=1		3,566	,000
department=2		0,000ᵃ	

Probability distribution:Multinomial
Link function:Cumulative logit

ᵃThis coefficient is set to zero because it is redundant.

In the random intercept model we have also commanded predicted values (variable 7) and predicted probabilities of having the predicted values as computed by the software (variables 5 and 6).

1	2	3	4	5	6	7 (variables)
0	1	1.00	1.00	0.224	0.895	1
0	1	1.00	2.00	0.224	0.895	1
0	1	2.00	3.00	0.241	0.903	1
0	1	1.00	4.00	0.224	0.895	1

(continued)

(continued)

1	2	3	4	5	6	7 (variables)
0	1	1.00	5.00	0.224	0.895	1
0	1	0.00	6.00	0.007	0.163	2
1	1	2.00	7.00	0.185	0.870	1
0	1	2.00	8.00	0.241	0.903	1
1	1	2.00	9.00	0.185	0.870	1
0	1	0.00	10.00	0.007	0.163	2

Variable 1: department
Variable 2: falloutofbed
Variable 3: agecat
Variable 4: patient_id
Variable 5: predicted probability of predicted value of target accounting the department score only
Variable 6: predicted probability of predicted value of target accounting both department and agecat scores
Variable 7: predicted value of target

Like automatic linear regression (see Chap. 7) and other generalized mixed linear models (see Chap. 9) random intercept models include the possibility to make XML files from the analysis, that can subsequently be used for making predictions about the chance of falling out of bed in future patients. However, SPSS uses here slightly different software called winRAR ZIP files that are "shareware". This means that you pay a small fee and be registered if you wish to use it. Note that winRAR ZIP files have an archive file format consistent of compressed data used by Microsoft since 2006 for the purpose of filing XML (eXtended Markup Language) files. They are only employable for a limited period of time like e.g. 40 days.

6.4 Conclusion

Generalized linear mixed models are suitable for analyzing data with multiple categorical variables. Random intercept versions of these models provide better sensitivity of testing than fixed intercept models.

6.5 Note

More information on statistical methods for analyzing data with categories is in the Chaps. 4 and 5 of this volume.

Chapter 7
Automatic Regression for Maximizing Linear Relationships (55 patients)

7.1 General Purpose

Automatic linear regression is in the Statistics Base add-on module SPSS version 19 and up. X-variables are automatically transformed in order to provide an improved data fit, and SPSS uses rescaling of time and other measurement values, outlier trimming, category merging and other methods for the purpose. This chapter is to assess whether automatic linear regression is helpful to obtain an improved precision of analysis of clinical trials.

7.2 Specific Scientific Question

In a clinical crossover trial an old laxative is tested against a new one. Numbers of stools per month is the outcome. The old laxative and the patients' age are the predictor variables. Does automatic linear regression provide better statistics of these data than traditional multiple linear regression does.

7.3 Data Example

Patno	Newtreat	Oldtreat	Age categories
1.00	24.00	8.00	2.00
2.00	30.00	13.00	2.00
3.00	25.00	15.00	2.00
4.00	35.00	10.00	3.00
5.00	39.00	9.00	3.00
6.00	30.00	10.00	3.00

(continued)

T. J. Cleophas and A. H. Zwinderman, *Machine Learning in Medicine—Cookbook Two*, SpringerBriefs in Statistics, DOI: 10.1007/978-3-319-07413-9_7, © The Author(s) 2014

(continued)

Patno	Newtreat	Oldtreat	Age categories
7.00	27.00	8.00	1.00
8.00	14.00	5.00	1.00
9.00	39.00	13.00	1.00
10.00	42.00	15.00	1.00

patno = patient number
newtreat = frequency of stools on a novel laxative
oldtreat = frequency of stools on an old laxative
agecategories = patients' age categories (1 = young, 2 = middle-age, 3 = old)

Only the first 10 patients of the 55 patients are shown above. The entire file is in extras.springer.com and is entitled "chap7automaticlinreg". We will first perform a standard multiple linear regression.

Command:

Analyze...Regression...Linear...Dependent: enter newtreat...Independent: enter oldtreat and agecategoriess...click OK.

Model Summary

Model	R	R Square	Adjusted R Square	Std. Error of the Estimate
1	,429ᵃ	,184	,133	9,28255

a. Predictors: (Constant), oldtreat, agecategories

ANOVAᵃ

Model		Sum of Squares	df	Mean Square	F	Sig.
1	Regression	622,869	2	311,435	3,614	,038ᵇ
	Residual	2757,302	32	86,166		
	Total	3380,171	34			

a. Dependent Variable: newtreat

b. Predictors: (Constant), oldtreat, agecategories

Coefficientsᵃ

Model		Unstandardized Coefficients		Standardized Coefficients	t	Sig.
		B	Std. Error	Beta		
1	(Constant)	20,513	5,137		3,993	,000
	agecategories	3,908	2,329	,268	1,678	,103
	oldtreat	,135	,065	,331	2,070	,047

a. Dependent Variable: newtreat

The above tables show that traditional linear regression is unable to demonstrate a significant effect of age and shows a borderline significant effect at p = 0.047 for the old laxative. Subsequently, an automatic linear regression is performed.

Command:

click Transform...click Random Number Generators...click Set Starting Point...click Fixed Value (20,00,000)...click OK...click Analyze....Regression.... Automatic Linear Regression...click Fields....newtreat drag to Target:...patientno drag to Analysis Weight:...oldtreat and agecategories drag to Fields:...click Build Options...click Objectives...mark Create a standard model...click Basics...mark Automatically prepare data...click Model Options...mark Save predicted values to the dataset....mark Export model....File name: type "exportautomaticlinreg"...click Browse and save the export file in the appropriate folder of your computer...click Run.

The underneath Automatic linear regression results show that the two predictors agecategories and oldtreat have been transformed, respectively into merged categories and a variable without outliers.

Automatic Data Preparation
Target: newtreat

Field	Role	Actions Taken
(agecategories_transformed)	Predictor	Merge categories to maximize association with target
(oldtreat_transformed)	Predictor	Trim outliers

If the original field name is X, then the transformed field is displayed as (X_transformed). The original field is excluded from the analysis and the transformed field is included instead.

An interactive graph shows the predictors as lines with thicknesses corresponding to their predictive power and the outcome in the form of a histogram with its best fit Gaussian pattern. Both of the predictors are now statistically very significant with a correlation coefficient at $p < 0.0001$, and regression coefficients at p-values of respectively 0.001 and 0.007.

Coefficients
Target: newtreat

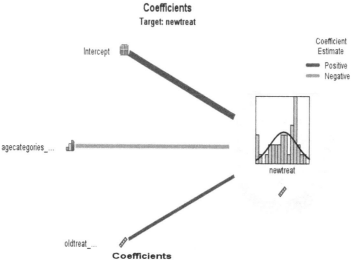

Coefficients
Target: newtreat

Model Term	Coefficient ▶	Sig.	Importance
Intercept	35,926	,000	
agecategories_transformed=0	-11,187	,001	0,609
agecategories_transformed=1	0,000ᵃ		0,609
oldtreat_transformed	0,209	,007	0,391

ᵃThis coefficient is set to zero because it is redundant.

Effects
Target: newtreat

Source	Sum of Squares	df	Mean Square	F	Sig.
Corrected Model ▶	1.289,960	2	644,980	9,874	,000
Residual	2.090,212	32	65,319		
Corrected Total	3.380,171	34			

Returning to the data view of the original data file, we now observe that SPSS has provided a novel variable with values for the new treatment as predicted from statistical model employed. They are pretty close to the real outcome values.

Patno	Newtreat	Oldtreat	Age categories	Predicted values
1.00	24.00	8.00	2.00	26.41
2.00	30.00	13.00	2.00	27.46
3.00	25.00	15.00	2.00	27.87
4.00	35.00	10.00	3.00	38.02
5.00	39.00	9.00	3.00	37.81
6.00	30.00	10.00	3.00	38.02
7.00	27.00	8.00	1.00	26.41
8.00	14.00	5.00	1.00	25.78
9.00	39.00	13.00	1.00	27.46
10.00	42.00	15.00	1.00	27.87

patno = patient number
newtreat = frequency of stools on a novel laxative
oldtreat = frequency of stools on an old laxative
agecategories = patients' age categories (1 = young, 2 = middle-age, 3 = old)

7.4 The Computer Teaches Itself to Make Predictions

The modeled regression coefficients are used to make predictions about future data using the Scoring Wizard and an XML (eXtended Markup Language) file (winRAR ZIP file) of the data file. Like random intercept models (see Chap. 6) and other generalized mixed linear models (see Chap. 9) automatic linear regression includes the possibility to make XML files from the analysis, that can subsequently be used for making outcome predictions in future patients. SPSS uses here software called winRAR ZIP files that are "shareware". This means that you pay a small fee and be registered if you wish to use it. Note that winRAR ZIP files have a archive file format consistent of compressed data used by Microsoft since 2006 for the purpose of filing XML files. They are only employable for a limited period of time like e.g. 40 days. Below the data of 9 future patients are given.

Newtreat	Oldtreat	Agecategory
	4.00	1.00
	13.00	1.00
	15.00	1.00
	15.00	1.00
	11.00	2.00
	80.00	2.00
	10.00	3.00
	18.00	2.00
	13.00	2.00

Enter the above data in a novel data file and command:

Utilities...click Scoring Wizard...click Browse....Open the appropriate folder with the XML file entitled "exportautomaticlinreg"...click on the latter and click Select...in Scoring Wizard double-click Next...mark Predicted Value...click Finish.

Newtreat	Oldtreat	Agecategory	Predictednewtreat
	4.00	1.00	25.58
	13.00	1.00	27.46
	15.00	1.00	27.87
	15.00	1.00	27.87
	11.00	2.00	27.04
	80.00	2.00	41.46
	10.00	3.00	38.02
	18.00	2.00	28.50
	13.00	2.00	27.46

In the data file SPSS has provided the novel variable as requested. The first patient with only four stools per month on the old laxative and young of age will have over 25 stools on the new laxative.

7.5 Conclusion

SPSS' automatic linear regression can be helpful to obtain an improved precision of analysis of clinical trials and provided in the example given better statistics than traditional multiple linear regression did.

7.6 Note

More background theoretical and mathematical information of linear regression is available in Statistics Applied to Clinical Studies 5th Edition, Chap. 14, entitled Linear regression basic approach, Chap. 15, Linear regression for assessing precision confounding interaction, Chap. 18, Regression modeling for improved precision, pp 161–176, 177–185, 219–225, Springer Heidelberg Germany, 2013, from the same authors.

Chapter 8
Simulation Models for Varying Predictors (9,000 Patients)

8.1 General Purpose

In medicine predictors are often varying, like, e.g., the numbers of complications and the days in hospital in patients with various conditions. This chapter is to assess, whether Monte Carlo simulation of the varying predictors can improve the outcome predictions.

8.2 Specific Scientific Question

The hospital costs for patients with heart infarction is supposed to be dependent on factors like patients' age, intensive care hours (ichours), numbers of complications. What percentage of patients will cost the hospital over 20,000 Euros, what percentage over 10,000. How will costs develop if the numbers of complications are reduced by 2 and the numbers of ichours by 20.

Instead of Traditional Means and Standard Deviations, Monte Carlo Simulations of the Input and Outcome Variables are Used to Model the Data. This Enhances Precision, Particularly, with Non-normal Data.

Age years	Complication number	Ic hours	Costs euros
48	7	36	5,488
66	7	57	8,346
75	7	67	6,976
72	6	45	5,691
60	6	58	3,637
84	9	54	16,369
74	8	54	11,349

(continued)

T. J. Cleophas and A. H. Zwinderman, *Machine Learning in Medicine—Cookbook Two*, SpringerBriefs in Statistics, DOI: 10.1007/978-3-319-07413-9_8, © The Author(s) 2014

(continued)

Age years	Complication number	Ic hours	Costs euros
42	9	26	10,213
71	7	49	6,474
73	10	35	30,018
53	8	37	7,632
79	6	46	6,538
50	10	39	13,797

Only the first 13 patients of this 9,000 patient hypothesized data file is shown. The entire data file is in extras.springer.com and is entitled "chap8simulation1.sav". SPSS 21 or 22 can be used. Start by opening the data file.

We will first perform a traditional linear regression with the first three variables as input and the fourth variable as outcome.

Command:

click Transform...click Random Number Generators...click Set Starting Point ...click Fixed Value (2,000,000)...click OK...click Analyze ...Regression...Linear...Dependent: costs...Independent: age, complication, ichours...click Save...click Browse...Select the desired folder in your computer...File name: enter "exportsimulation"...click Save...click Continue...click OK.

In the output sheets it is observed that all of the predictors are statistically very significant. Also a PMML (predictive model markup language) document, otherwise called XML (eXtended Markup Language) document has been produced and filed in your computer entitled "exportsimulation".

Coefficients[a]

Model		Unstandardized coefficients		Standardized coefficients	t	Sig.
		B	Std. error	Beta		
1	(Constant)	−28570.977	254.044		−112.465	0.000
	age (years)	202.403	2.767	0.318	73.136	0.000
	complications (n)	4022.405	21.661	0.807	185.696	0.000
	ichours (hours)	−111.241	2.124	−0.227	−52.374	0.000

a. Dependent Variable: cost (Euros)

We will now perform the Monte Carlo simulation.

Command: Analyze...Simulation...click Select SPSS Model File...click Continue...in Look in: select folder with "exportsimulation.xml" file...click Open...–click Simulation Fields...click Fit All...click Save...mark Save the plan file for this simulation...click Browse...in Look in: select the appropriate folder for storage of a simulation plan document and entitle it, e.g., "splan"...click Save...click Run.

In the output the underneath interactive probability density graph is exhibited. After double-clicking the vertical lines can be moved and corresponding areas under the curve percentages are shown.

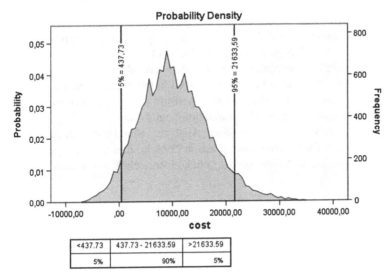

<437.73	437.73 - 21633.59	>21633.59
5%	90%	5%

Overall 90 % of the heart attacks patients will cost the hospital between 440 and 21.630 Euros. In the graph click Chart Options...in View click Histogram...click Continue.

The histogram below is displayed. Again the vertical lines can be moved as desired. It can, e.g., be observed that, around, 7.5 % of the heart attack patients will cost the hospital over 20.000 Euros, around 50 % of them will cost over 10.000 Euros.

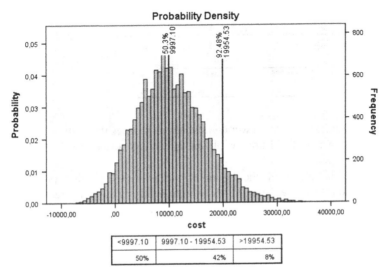

<9997.10	9997.10 - 19954.53	>19954.53
50%	42%	8%

Monte Carlo can also be used to answer questions like "What will happen to costs, if the numbers of complications are reduced by two or the ichours are reduced by 20". For that purpose we will use the original data file entitled "chap8 simulation1.sav" again. Also the document entitled "splan" which contains software syntax for performing a simulation is required.

Open "chap8simulation1.sav" and command: Transform...Compute Variable...in Numeric Expression enter "complications" from the panel below Numeric Expressions enter "-" and "2"...in Target Variable type complications....click OK...in Change existing variable click OK.

In the data file all of the values of the variable "complications" have now been reduced by 2. This transformed data file is saved in the desired folder and entitled e.g. "chap8simulation2.sav". We will now perform a Monte Carlo simulation of this transformed data file using the simulation plan "splan".

In "chap8simulation2.sav" command: Analyze...Simulation...click Open an Existing Simulation Plan...click Continue...in Look in: find the appropriate folder in your computer...click "splan.splan"...click Open...click Simulation...click Fit All...click Run.

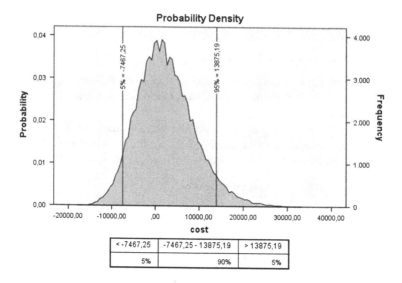

< -7467,25	-7467,25 - 13875,19	> 13875,19
5%	90%	5%

The above graph shows that fewer complications reduces the costs, e.g., 5 % of the patients cost over 13.875 Euros, while the same class costed over 21.633 Euros before.

What about the effect of the hours in the ic unit. For that purpose, in "chap8simulation1.sav" perform the same commands as shown directly above, and transform the ichours variable by −20 h. The transformed document can be named "chap8simulation3.sav" and saved. The subsequent simulation procedure in this data file using again "splan.splan" produces the underneath output.

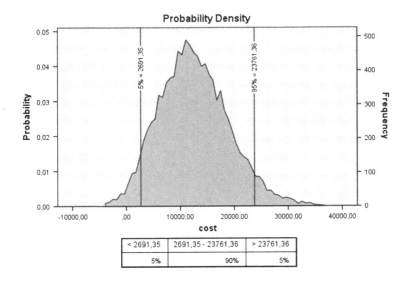

It is observed that the costs are now not reduced, but rather somewhat increased with 5 % of the patients costing over 23.761 Euros instead of 21.633. This would make sense, nonetheless, because it is sometimes assumed by hospital managers that the reduction of stay-days in hospital is accompanied with more demanding type of care (Statistics Applied to Clinical Studies, 5th Edition, Chap. 44, Clinical data where variability is more important than averages, pp 487–498, Springer Heidelberg Germany, 2012).

8.3 Conclusion

Monte Carlo simulations of inputs where variability is more important than means can model outcome distributions with increased precision. This is, particularly, so with non-normal data.

Also questions like "how will hospital costs develop, if the numbers of complications are reduced by 2 or numbers of hours in the intensive care unit reduced by 20, can be answered.

8.4 Note

More background, theoretical and mathematical information of Monte Carlo simulation is provided in Statistics Applied to Clinical Studies, 5th Edition, Chap. 44, Clinical data where variability is more important than averages, pp 487–498, Springer Heidelberg Germany, 2012, from the same authors as the current publication.

Chapter 9
Generalized Linear Mixed Models for Outcome Prediction from Mixed Data (20 Patients)

9.1 General Purpose

To assess whether generalized linear mixed models can be used to train clinical samples with both fixed and random effects about individual future patients.

9.2 Specific Scientific Question

In a parallel-group study of two treatments, each patient was measured weekly for 5 weeks. As repeated measures in one patient are more similar than unrepeated ones, a random interaction effect between week and patient was assumed.

9.3 Example

In a parallel-group study of two cholesterol reducing compounds, patients were measured weekly for 5 weeks. As repeated measures in one patient are more similar than unrepeated ones, we assumed that a random interaction variable between week and patient would appropriately adjust this effect.

Patient_id	Week	Hdl-cholesterol (mmol/l)	Treatment (0 or 1)
1	1	1.66	0
1	2	1.62	0
1	3	1.57	0
1	4	1.52	0
1	5	1.50	0
2	1	1.69	0

(continued)

T. J. Cleophas and A. H. Zwinderman, *Machine Learning in Medicine—Cookbook Two*, SpringerBriefs in Statistics, DOI: 10.1007/978-3-319-07413-9_9, © The Author(s) 2014

(continued)

Patient_id	Week	Hdl-cholesterol (mmol/l)	Treatment (0 or 1)
2	2	1.71	0
2	3	1.60	0
2	4	1.55	0
2	5	1.56	0

Only the first two patients of the data file is shown. The entire file entitled "chap9fixedandrandomeffects" is in extras.springer.com. We will try and develop a mixed model (mixed means a model with both fixed and random predictors) for testing the data. Also, SPSS will be requested to produce a ZIP (compressed file that can be unzipped) file from the intervention study, which could then be used for making predictions about cholesterol values in future patients treated similarly. We will start by opening the intervention study's data file.

Command:

Click Transform...click Random Number Generators...click Set Starting Point...click Fixed Value (20,00,000)...click OK...click Analyze...Mixed Linear...Generalized Mixed Linear Models...click Data Structure...click left mouse and drag patient_id to Subjects part of the canvas...click left mouse and drag week to Repeated Measures part of the canvas...click Fields and Effects...click Target...check that the variable outcome is already in the Target window...check that Linear model is marked...click Fixed Effects...drag treatment and week to Effect builder....click Random Effects....click Add Block....click Add a custom term... move week*treatment (* is symbol multiplication and interaction) to the Custom term window...click Add term...click OK...click Model Options...click Save Fields...mark Predicted Values...click Export model... type exportfixedandrandom ...click Browse...in the appropriate folder enter in File name: mixed...click Run.

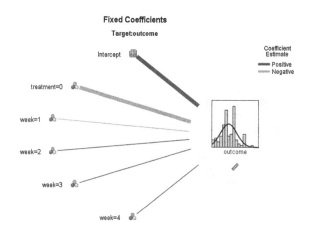

Source	F	df1	df2	Sig.
Corrected Model ▼	5,027	5	94	,000
treatment	23,722	1	94	,000
week	0,353	4	94	,841

Probability distribution:Normal
Link function:Identity

In the output sheet a graph is observed with the mean and standard errors of the outcome value displayed with the best fit Gaussian curve. The F-value of 23.722 indicates that one treatment is very significantly better than the other with $p < 0.0001$. The thickness of the lines are a measure for level of significance, and so the significance of the 5 week is very thin and thus very weak. Week 5 is not shown. It is redundant, because it means absence of the other 4 weeks. If you click at the left bottom of the graph panel, a table comes up providing similar information in written form. The effect of the interaction variable is not shown, but implied in the analysis.

If we return to the data file page, we will observe that the software has produced a predicted value for each actually measured cholesterol value. The predicted and actual values are very much the same.

We will now use the ZIP file to make predictions about cholesterol values in future patients treated similarly.

Week	Treatment	Patient_id
1	0	21
2	0	21
3	0	21
4	0	21
5	0	21
1	1	22
2	1	22
3	1	22
4	1	22
5	1	22

Command:
Click Utilities...click Scoring Wizard...click Browse...click Select...Folder: enter the mixed ZIP file entitled "exportfixedandrandom"...click Select...in Scoring Wizard click Next...click Finish.

In the data file now the predicted cholesterol values are given.

Week	Treatment	Patient_id	Predicted cholesterol
1	0	21	1.88
2	0	21	1.96
3	0	21	1.94
4	0	21	1.91
5	0	21	1.89
1	1	22	2.12
2	1	22	2.20
3	1	22	2.18
4	1	22	2.15
5	1	22	2.13

9.4 Conclusion

The module Generalized mixed linear models provides the possibility to handle both fixed and random effects, and is, therefore appropriate to adjust data with repeated measures and presumably a strong correlation between the repeated measures. Also individual future patients treated similarly can be assessed for predicted cholesterol values using a ZIP file.

9.5 Note

More background theoretical and mathematical information of models with both fixed and random variables is given in:

1. Machine Learning in Medicine Part One Machine Learning in Medicine Part One, Chap. 6, Mixed linear models, pp 65–76, 2013,
2. Statistics Applied to Clinical Studies, 5th Edition Statistics Applied to Clinical Studies, 5th Edition, Chap. 56, Advanced analysis of variance, random effects and mixed effects models, pp 607–618, 2012,
3. SPSS for Starters Part One SPSS for Starters Part One, Chap. 7, Mixed models, pp 25–29, 2010, and,
4. Machine Learning in Medicine Part Three Machine Learning in Medicine Part Three, Chap. 9, Random Effects, pp 81–94, 2013.

All of these references are from the same authors and have been edited by Springer Heidelberg Germany.

Chapter 10
Two-stage Least Squares (35 Patients)

10.1 General Purpose

The two stage least squares method assumes that the independent variable (x-variable) is problematic, meaning that it is somewhat uncertain. An additional variable can be argued to provide relevant information about the problematic variable, and is, therefore, called instrumental variable, and included in the analysis.

10.2 Primary Scientific Question

Non-compliance is a predictor of drug efficacy. Counseling causes improvement of patients' compliance and, therefore, indirectly improves the outcome drug efficacy.

y = outcome variable (drug efficacy)
x = problematic variable (non-compliance)
z = instrumental variable (counseling).

With two stage least squares the underneath stages are assessed.

1st stage
x = intercept + regression coefficient times z

T. J. Cleophas and A. H. Zwinderman, *Machine Learning in Medicine—Cookbook Two*, SpringerBriefs in Statistics, DOI: 10.1007/978-3-319-07413-9_10, © The Author(s) 2014

With the help of the calculated intercept and regression coefficient from the above simple linear regression analysis improved x-values are calculated e.g. for patient 1:

$x_{improved}$ = intercept + regression coefficient times 8 = 27.68
2nd stage
y = intercept + regression coefficient times $x_{improved}$

10.3 Example

Patients' non-compliance is a factor notoriously affecting the estimation of drug efficacy. An example is given of a simple evaluation study that assesses the effect of non-compliance (pills not used) on the outcome, the efficacy of a novel laxative with numbers of stools per month as efficacy estimator (the y-variable). The data of the first 10 of the 35 patients are in the table below. The entire data file is in extras.springer.com, and is entitled "chap10twostageleastsquares".

Patient no	Instrumental variable (z)	Problematic predictor (x)	Outcome (y)
	Frequency counseling	Pills not used (non-compliance)	Efficacy estimator of new laxative (stools/month)
1.	8	25	24
2.	13	30	30
3.	15	25	25
4.	14	31	35
5.	9	36	39
6.	10	33	30
7.	8	22	27
8.	5	18	14
9.	13	14	39
10.	15	30	42

SPSS version 19 and up can be used for analysis. It uses the term explanatory variable for the problematic variable. Start by opening the data file. Then, command:

Analyze....Regression....2 Stage Least Squares....Dependent: therapeutic efficacy....Explanatory: non-compliance.... Instrumental: counseling ...OK.

Model Description

		Type of variable
Equation 1	y	dependent
	x	predictor
	z	instrumental

ANOVA

		Sum of Squares	Df	Mean Square	F	Sig.
Equation 1	Regression	1408.040	1	1408.040	4.429	0.043
	Residual	10490.322	33	317.889		
	Total	11898.362	34			

Coefficients

		Unstandardized coefficients		Beta	t	Sig.
		B	Std. error			
Equation 1	(Constant)	−49.778	37.634		−1.323	0.195
	x	2.675	1.271	1.753	2.105	0.043

The result is shown above. The non-compliance adjusted for counseling is a statistically significant predictor of laxative efficacy with p = 0.043. This p-value has been automatically been adjusted for multiple testing. When we test the model without the help of the instrumental variable counseling the p-value is larger and the effect is no more statistically significant as shown underneath.

Command: Analyze...Regression...Linear...Dependent: therapeutic efficacy... Independent: non-compliance...OK.

ANOVA[b]

Model		Sum of squares	Df	Mean square	F	Sig.
1	Regression	334.482	1	334.482	3.479	0.071[a]
	Residual	3172.489	33	96.136		
	Total	3506.971	34			

[a] Predictors: (Constant), non-compliance
[b] Dependent Variable: drug efficacy

Coefficients[a]

		Unstandardized coefficients		Standardized coefficients		
		B	Std. error	Beta	t	Sig.
1	(Constant)	15.266	7.637		1.999	0.054
	non-compliance	0.471	0.253	0.309	1.865	0.071

a. Dependent Variable: drug efficacy

10.4 Conclusion

Two stage least squares with counseling as instrumental variable was more sensitive than simple linear regression with laxative efficacy as outcome and non-compliance as predictor. We should add that two stage least squares is at risk of overestimating the precision of the outcome, if the analysis is not adequately adjusted for multiple testing. However, in SPSS automatic adjustment for the purpose has been performed. The example is the simplest version of the procedure. And, multiple explanatory and instrumental variables can be included in the models.

10.5 Note

More background theoretical and mathematical information of two stage least squares analyses is given in Machine Learning in Medicine Part Two, Two-stage least squares, pp 9–15, Springer Heidelberg Germany, 2013, from the same authors.

Chapter 11
Autoregressive Models for Longitudinal Data (120 Mean Monthly Records of a Population of Diabetic Patients)

11.1 General Purpose

Time series are encountered in every field of medicine. Traditional tests are unable to assess trends, seasonality, change points and the effects of multiple predictors like treatment modalities simultaneously. To assess whether autoregressive integrated moving average (ARIMA) methods are able to do all of that.

11.2 Specific Scientific Question

Monthly HbA1c levels in patients with diabetes type II are a good estimator for adequate diabetes control, and have been demonstrated to be seasonal with higher levels in the winter. A large patient population was followed for 10 year. The mean values are in the data. This chapter is to assess whether longitudinal summary statistics of a population can be used for the effects of seasons and treatment changes on populations with chronic diseases.

Note:

No conclusion can here be drawn about individual patients. Autoregressive models can also be applied with data sets of individual patients, and with multiple outcome variables like various health outcomes.

T. J. Cleophas and A. H. Zwinderman, *Machine Learning in Medicine—Cookbook Two*, SpringerBriefs in Statistics, DOI: 10.1007/978-3-319-07413-9_11, © The Author(s) 2014

11.3 Example

The underneath data are from the first year's observation data of the above diabetic patient data. The entire data file is in extras.springer.com, and is entitled "chap11arimafile".

Date	HbA1	Nurse	Doctor	Phone	Self	Meeting
01/01/1989	11.00	8.00	7.00	3	22	2
02/01/1989	10.00	8.00	9.00	3	27	2
03/01/1989	17.00	8.00	7.00	2	30	3
04/01/1989	7.00	8.00	9.00	2	29	2
05/01/1989	7.00	9.00	7.00	2	23	2
06/01/1989	10.00	8.00	9.00	3	27	2
07/01/1989	9.00	8.00	8.00	3	27	2
08/01/1989	10.00	8.00	7.00	3	30	2
09/01/1989	12.00	8.00	8.00	4	27	2
10/01/1989	13.00	9.00	11.00	3	32	2
11/01/1989	14.00	9.00	7.00	3	29	2
12/01/1989	23.00	10.00	11.00	5	39	3
01/01/1990	12.00	8.00	7.00	4	23	2
02/01/1990	8.00	8.00	6.00	2	25	3

Date = date of observation
HbA1 = mean HbA1c of diabetes population
nurse = mean number of diabetes nurse visits
doctor = mean number of doctor visits
phone = mean number of phone visits
self = mean number of self-controls
meeting = mean number of patient educational meetings

We will first assess the observed values along the time line. The analysis is performed using SPSS statistical software.

Command: analyze....Forecast....Sequence   Charts....Variables: enter HbA1c....Time Axis Labels: enter Date....OK.

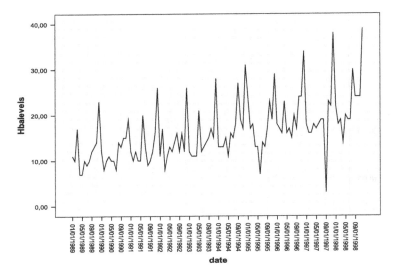

The above output sheets show the observed data. There are (1) numerous peaks, which are (2) approximately equally sized, and (3) there is an upward trend: (2) suggests periodicity which was expected from the seasonal pattern of HbA1c values, (3) is also expected, it suggests increasing HbA1c after several years due to beta-cell failure. Finally (4), there are several peaks that are not part of the seasonal pattern, and could be due to outliers.

ARIMA (autoregressive integrated moving average methodology) is used for modeling this complex data pattern. It uses the Export Modeler for outlier detection, and produces for the purpose XML (eXtended Markup Language) files for prediction modeling of future data.

Command:

Analyze....Forecast....Time Series Modeler....Dependent Variables: enter HbA1c....Independent Variables: enter nurse, doctor, phone, self control, and patient meeting....click Methods: Expert Modeler....click Criteria....Click Outlier Table....Select automatically ....Click Statistics Table....Select Parameter Estimates....mark Display forecasts....click Plots table....click Series, Observed values, Fit values....click Save....Predicted Values: mark Save....Export XML File: click Browse....various folders in your PC come up....in "File Name" of the appropriate folder enter "exportarima"....click Save....click Continue....click OK.

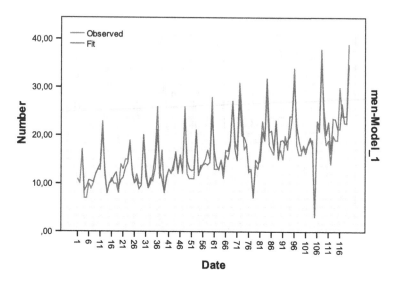

The above graph shows that a good fit of the observed data is given by the ARIMA model, and that an adequate predictive model is provided. The upward trend is in agreement with beta-cell failure after several years.

The underneath table shows that 3 significant predictors have been identified. Also the goodness of fit of the ARIMA (p, d, q) model is given, where p = number of lags, d = the trend (one upward trend means d = 1), and q = number of moving averages (= 0 here). Both Stationary R square, and Ljung-Box tests are insignificant. A significant test would have meant poor fit. In our example, there is an adequate fit, but the model has identified no less than 7 outliers. Phone visits, nurse visits, and doctor visits were significant predictors at $p < 0.0001$, while self control and educational patient meetings were not so. All of the outliers are significantly more distant from the ARIMA model than could happen by chance. All of the p-values were very significant with $p < 0.001$ and <0.0001.

Model statistics						
Model	Number of predictors	Model fit statistics	Liung-Box Q(18)			Number of outliers
		Stationary R- squared	Statistics	DF	Sig.	
men-Model_1	3	0.898	17.761	18	0.471	7

ARIMA model parameters								
					Estimate	SE	t	Siq.
men-Model_1	Men	Natural Log	Constant		−2.828	0.456	−6.207	0.000
	Phone	Natural Log	Numerator	LagO	0.569	0.064	8.909	0.000

(continued)

(continued)

ARIMA model parameters

					Estimate	SE	t	Siq.
Nurse	Natural Log	Numerator		LagO	1.244	0.118	10.585	0.000
Doctor	Natural Log	Numerator		LagO	0.310	0.077	4.046	0.000
				Lag 1	−0.257	0.116	−2.210	0.029
				Lag 2	−0.196	0.121	−1.616	0.109
			Denominator	Lag 1	0.190	0.304	0.623	0.535

Outliers

			Estimate	SE	t	Sig.
men-Model_1	3	Additive	0.769	0.137	5.620	0.000
	30	Additive	0.578	0.138	4.198	0.000
	53	Additive	0.439	0.135	3.266	0.001
	69	Additive	0.463	0.135	3.439	0.001
	78	Additive	−0.799	0.138	−5.782	0.000
	88	Additive	0.591	0.134	4.409	0.000
	105	Additive	−1.771	0.134	−13.190	0.000

When returning to the data view screen, we will observe that SPSS has added HbA1 values (except for the first two dates due to lack of information) as a novel variable. The predicted values are pretty similar to the measured values, supporting the adequacy of the model.

We will now apply the XML file and the Apply Models modus for making predictions about HbA1 values in the next 6 months, assuming that the significant variables nurse, doctor, phone are kept constant at their overall means.

First add the underneath data to the original data file and rename the file, e.g., "chap11arimafile2", and store it at an appropriate folder in your computer.

Date	HbA1	Nurse	Doctor	Phone	Self	Meeting
01/01/1999		10.00	8.00	4.00		
01/02/1999		10.00	8.00	4.00		
01/03/1999		10.00	8.00	4.00		
01/04/1999		10.00	8.00	4.00		
01/05/1999		10.00	8.00	4.00		
01/06/1999		10.00	8.00	4.00		

Then open "chap11arimafile2.sav and command:

Analyze….click Apply Models….click Reestimate from data….click First case after end of estimation period through a specified date….Observation: enter 01/06/1999….click Statistics: click Display Forecasts….click Save: Predicted Values mark Save….click OK.

The underneath table shows the predicted HbA1 values for the next 6 months and their upper and lower confidence limits (UCL and LCL).

Forecast							
Model		121	122	123	124	125	126
HbA1-Model_1	Forecast	17.69	17.30	16.49	16.34	16.31	16.30
	UCL	22.79	22.28	21.24	21.05	21.01	21.00
	LCL	13.49	13.19	12.58	12.46	12.44	12.44

For each model, forecasts start after the last non-missing in the range of the requested estimation period, and end at the last period for which non-missing values of all the predictors are available or at the end date of the requested forecast period, whichever is earlier

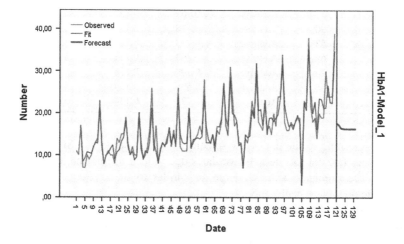

Also a graph of the HbA1 pattern after the estimation period is given as shown in the above graph. When returning to the data view of the arimafile2, we will observe that SPSS has added the predicted values as a novel variable.

Date	HbA1	Nurse	Doctor	Phone	Self	Meeting	Modeled HbA1	Predicted HbA1
07/01/1998	19.00	11.00	8.00	5.00	28.00	4.00	21.35	21.35
08/01/1998	30.00	12.00	9.00	4.00	27.00	5.00	21.31	21.31
09/01/1998	24.00	13.00	8.00	5.00	30.00	5.00	26.65	26.65
10/01/1998	24.00	12.00	10.00	4.00	28.00	6.00	22.59	22.59
11/01/1998	24.00	11.00	8.00	5.00	26.00	5.00	22.49	22.49
12/01/1998	39.00	15.00	10.00	5.00	37.00	7.00	34.81	34.81
01/01/1999		10.00	8.00	4.00				17.69
01/02/1999		10.00	8.00	4.00				17.30
01/03/1999		10.00	8.00	4.00				16.49
01/04/1999		10.00	8.00	4.00				16.34

(continued)

(continued)

Date	HbA1	Nurse	Doctor	Phone	Self	Meeting	Modeled HbA1	Predicted HbA1
01/05/1999		10.00	8.00	4.00				16.31
01/06/1999		10.00	8.00	4.00				16.30

Modeled HbA1 = calculated HbA1 values from the above arima model
Predicted HbA1 = the predicted HbA1 values using the XML file for future dates

11.4 Conclusion

Autoregressive integrated moving average methods are appropriate for assessing trends, seasonality, and change points in a time series. In the example given no conclusion can be drawn about individual patients. Autoregressive models can, however, also be applied for data sets of individual patients. Also as a multivariate methodology it is appropriate for multiple instead of a single outcome variable like various health outcomes.

11.5 Note

More background theoretical and mathematical information of autoregressive models for longitudinal data is in Machine Learning in Medicine Part Two, Multivariate analysis of time series, pp 139–154, Springer Heidelberg Germany, 2013, from the same authors.

Part III
Rules Models

Chapter 12
Item Response Modeling for Analyzing Quality of Life with Better Precision (1,000 Patients)

12.1 General Purpose

Item response tests are goodness of fit tests for analyzing the item scores of intelligence tests, and they perform better for the purpose than traditional tests, based on reproducibility measures, do. Like intelligence, quality of life is a multidimensional construct, and may, therefore, be equally suitable for item response modeling.

12.2 Primary Scientific Question

Can quality of life data be analyzed through item response modeling, and provide more sensitivity than classical linear models do?

12.3 Example

As an example we will analyze the 5-items of a mobility-domain of a quality of life (QOL) battery for patients with coronary artery disease in a group of 1,000 patients. Instead of 5 many more items can be included. However, for the purpose of simplicity we will use only 5 items: the domain mobility in a quality of life battery was assessed by answering "yes or no" to experienced difficulty (1) while climbing stair, (2) on short distances, (3) on long distances, (4) on light household work, (5) on heavy household work. In the underneath table the data of 1,000 patients are summarized. These data can be fitted into a standard normal Gaussian frequency distribution curve (see underneath figure). From it, it can be seen that the items used here are more adequate for demonstrating low quality of life than they are for demonstrating high quality of life, but, nonetheless, an entire Gaussian distribution can be extrapolated from the data given. The lack of histogram bars on the right side of the Gaussian curve suggests that more high quality of life items in

T. J. Cleophas and A. H. Zwinderman, *Machine Learning in Medicine—Cookbook Two*, SpringerBriefs in Statistics, DOI: 10.1007/978-3-319-07413-9_12, © The Author(s) 2014

the questionnaire would be welcome in order to improve the fit of the histogram into the Gaussian curve. Yet it is interesting to observe that, even with a limited set of items, already a fairly accurate frequency distribution pattern of all quality of life levels of the population is obtained.

No. response pattern	Response pattern (1 = yes, 2 = no) to items 1–5	Observed frequencies
1	11,111	4
2	11,112	7
3	11,121	3
4	11,122	12
5	11,211	2
6	11,212	2
7	11,221	4
8	11,222	5
9	12,111	2
10	12,112	9
11	12,121	1
12	12,122	17
13	12,211	1
14	12,212	4
15	12,221	3
16	12,222	16
17	21,111	11
18	21,112	30
19	21,121	15
20	21,122	21
21	21,211	4
22	21,212	29
23	21,221	16
24	21,222	81
25	22,111	17
26	22,112	57
27	22,121	22
28	22,122	174
29	22,211	12
30	22,212	62
31	22,221	29
32	22,222	263

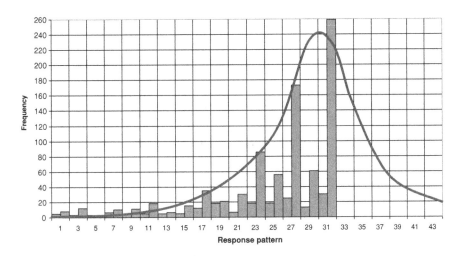

The LTA-2 (Latent Trait Analysis—2) free software program is used (Uebersax J. Free Software LTA (latent trait analysis)—2 (with binary items), 2006, www.john-uebersax.com/stat/Ital.htm). The data file entitled "chap12itemresponse-modeling" is available in extras.springer.com. We enter the data file by the traditional copy and paste commands.

Command:

Gaussian error model for IRF (Instrument Response Function) shape…chi-square goodness of fit for Fit Statistics…. Frequency table….EAP score table.

The software program calculates the quality of life scores of the different response patterns as EAP (Expected Ability a Posteriori) scores. These scores can be considered as the z-values of a normal Gaussian curve, meaning that the associated area under curve (AUC) of the Gaussian curve is an estimate of the level of quality of life.

There is, approximately,

a 50 % quality of life level with an EAP score of 0,

a 35 % QOL level with an EAP score of −1 (standard deviations),

a 2.5 % QOL level with an EAP score of −2

a 85 % QOL level with an EAP score of +1

a 97.5 % QOL level with an EAP score of +2

No.response Pattern	Response pattern (1 = yes, 2 = no) to items 1 to 5	EAP scores (SDs)	AUCs (QOL levels) (%)	Classical Scores (0-5)
1	11,111	−1.8315	3.4	0
2	11,112	−1.4425	7.5	1
3	11121	−1.4153	7.8	1
4	11,122	−1.0916	15.4	2
5	11,211	−1.2578	10.4	1
6	11,212	−0.8784	18.9	2
7	11,221	−0.8600	19.4	2
8	11,222	−0.4596	32.3	3
9	12,111	−1.3872	8.2	1
10	12,112	−0.9946	16.1	2
11	12,121	−0.9740	16.6	2
12	12,122	−0.5642	28.8	3
13	12,211	−0.8377	20.1	2
14	12,212	−0.4389	33.0	3
15	12,221	−0.4247	33.4	3
16	12,222	0.0074	50.4	4
17	21,111	−1.3501	8.9	1
18	21,112	−0.9381	17.4	2
19	21,121	−0.9172	17.9	2
20	21,122	−0.4866	31.2	3
21	21,211	−0.7771	21.8	2
22	21,212	−0.3581	35.9	3
23	21,221	−0.3439	36.7	3
24	21,222	0.1120	54.4	4
25	22,111	−0.8925	18.7	2
26	22,112	−0.4641	32.3	3
27	22,121	−0.4484	32.6	3
28	22,122	0.0122	50.4	4
29	22,211	−0.3231	37.5	3
30	22212	0.1322	55.2	4
31	22,221	0.1433	55.6	4
32	22,222	0.6568	74.5	5

EAP = expected ability a posteriori; QOL = quality of life

In the above table the EAP scores per response pattern is given as well as the
AUC (= quality of life level) values as calculated by the software program are
given. In the fourth column the classical score is given ranging from 0 (no yes
answers) to five (five yes answers). Unlike the classical scores, running from 0 to
100 %, the item scores are more precise and vary from 3.4 to 74.5 % with an
overall mean score, by definition, of 50 %. The item response model produce an
adequate fit for the data as demonstrated by chi-square goodness of fit values/
degrees of freedom of 0.86. What is even more important, is, that we have 32

different QOL scores instead of no more than 5 as observed with the classical score method. With 6 items the numbers of scores would even rise to 64. The interpretation is: the higher the score, the better the quality of life.

12.4 Conclusion

Quality of life assessments can be analyzed through item response modeling, and provide more sensitivity than classical linear models do.

12.5 Note

More background theoretical and mathematical information of item response modeling is given in Machine Learning in Medicine Part One, Chap. 8, Item Response Modeling, pp 87–98, edited by Springer Heidelberg Germany, 2012, from the same authors. In the current chapter the LTA-2 the free software program is used (Uebersax J. Free Software LTA (latent trait analysis) -2 (with binary items), 2006, www.john-uebersax.com/stat/Ital.htm).

Chapter 13
Survival Studies with Varying Risks of Dying (50 and 60 Patients)

13.1 General Purpose

Patients' predictors of survival may change across time, because people may change their lifestyles. Standard statistical methods do not allow adjustments for time-dependent predictors. Time-dependent Cox regression has been introduced as a method adequate for the purpose.

13.2 Primary Scientific Questions

Predictors of survival may change across time, e.g., the effect of smoking, cholesterol, and increased blood pressure on cardiovascular disease, and patients' frailty in oncology research.

13.3 Examples

13.3.1 Cox Regression with a Time-Dependent Predictor

The level of LDL cholesterol is a strong predictor of cardiovascular survival. However, in a survival study virtually no one will die from elevated values in the first decade of observation. LDL cholesterol may be, particularly, a killer in the second decade of observation. The Cox regression model is not appropriate for analyzing the effect of LDL cholesterol on survival, because it assumes that the relative hazard of dying is the same in the first, second and third decade. If you want to analyze such data, an extended Cox regression model allowing for non-proportional hazards can be applied, and is available in SPSS statistical software. In the underneath example the first 10 of 60 patients are given. They were followed for 30 years for the occurrence of a cardiovascular event. Each row represents a patient, the columns are the patient characteristics, otherwise called the variables.

Variable (Var)					
1	2	3	4	5	6
1.00	1	0	65.00	0.00	2.00
1.00	1	0	66.00	0.00	2.00
2.00	1	0	73.00	0.00	2.00
2.00	1	0	54.00	0.00	2.00
2.00	1	0	46.00	0.00	2.00
2.00	1	0	37.00	0.00	2.00
2.00	1	0	54.00	0.00	2.00
2.00	1	0	66.00	0.00	2.00
2.00	1	0	44.00	0.00	2.00
3.00	0	0	62.00	0.00	2.00

Var 00001 = follow-up period (years) (Var = variable)
Var 00002 = event (0 or 1, event or lost for follow-up = censored)
Var 00003 = treatment modality (0 = treatment-1, 1 = treatment-2)
Var 00004 = age (years)
Var 00005 = gender (0 or 1, male or female)
Var 00006 = LDL-cholesterol (0 or 1, < 3.9 or > = 3.9 mmol/l)

The entire data file is in extras.springer.com, and is entitled "Chap13survivalvaryingrisks". Start by opening the file. First, a usual Cox regression is performed with LDL-cholesterol as predictor of survival (var = variable).

Command: Analyze....survival....Cox regression....time: follow months.... status: var 2....define event (1)....Covariates....categorical: elevated LDL-cholesterol (Var 00006) => categorical variables....continue....plots.... survival => ....hazard....continue....OK.

Variables in the Equation

	B	SE	Wald	df	Sig.	Exp(B)
Var00006	−0.482	0.307	2.462	1	0.117	0.618

Variables in the Equation

	B	SE	Wald	df	Sig.	Exp(B)
T_COV_	−0.131	0.303	15.904	1	0.000	0.877

The upper table shows that elevated LDL-cholesterol is not a significant predictor of survival with a p-value as large as 0.117 and a hazard ratio of 0.618. In order to assess, whether elevated LDL-cholesterol adjusted for time has an effect on survival, a time-dependent Cox regression will be performed as shown in the above lower table. For that purpose the time-dependent covariate is defined as a function of both the variable time (called " T_" in SPSS) and the LDL-cholesterol-variable, while using the product of the two. This product is applied as the "time-dependent predictor of survival, and a usual Cox model is, subsequently, performed (Cov = covariate).

Command: Analyze....survival....Cox w/Time-Dep Cov....Compute Time-Dep Cov....Time (T_) => in box Expression for T_Cov....add the sign * ....add the LDL-cholesterol variable....model....time: follow months....status: var 00002....?: define event:1....continue....T_Cov => in box covariates....OK.

The above lower table shows that elevated LDL-cholesterol after adjustment for differences in time is a highly significant predictor of survival. If we look at the actual data of the file, we will observe that, overall, the LDL-cholesterol variable is not an important factor. But, if we look at the LDL-cholesterol levels of the three decades separately, then it is observed that something very special is going on: in the first decade virtually no one with elevated LDL-cholesterol dies. In the second decade virtually everyone with an elevated LDL-cholesterol does: LDL cholesterol seems to be particularly a killer in the second decade. Then, in the third decade other reasons for dying seem to have occurred.

13.3.2 Cox Regression with a Segmented Time-Dependent Predictor

Some variables may have different values at different time periods. For example, elevated blood pressure may be, particularly, harmful not after decades but at the very time-point it is highest. The blood pressure is highest in the first and third decade of the study. However, in the second decade it is mostly low, because the patients were adequately treated at that time. For the analysis we have to use the socalled logical expressions. They take the value 1, if the time is true, and 0, if false. Using a series of logical expressions, we can create our time-dependent predictor, that can, then, be analyzed by the usual Cox model. In the underneath example 11 of 60 patients are given. The entire data file is in extras.springer.com, and is entitled "Chap. 13 survivalvaryingrisks2" The patients were followed for 30 years for the occurrence of a cardiovascular event. Each row represents again a patient, the columns are the patient characteristics.

(continued)

Var 1	2	3	4	5	6	7
Var 1	2	3	4	5	6	7
7.00	1	76	0.00	133.00		
9.00	1	76	0.00	134.00		
9.00	1	65	0.00	143.00		
11.00	1	54	0.00	134.00	110.00	
12.00	1	34	0.00	143.00	111.00	
14.00	1	45	0.00	135.00	110.00	
16.00	1	56	1.00	123.00	103.00	
17.00	1	67	1.00	133.00	107.00	
18.00	1	86	1.00	134.00	108.00	
30.00	1	75	1.00	134.00	102.00	134.00
30.00	1	65	1.00	132.00	121.00	126.00

Var 00001 = follow-up period years (Var = variable)
Var 00002 = event (0 or 1, event or lost for follow-up = censored)
Var 00003 = age (years)
Var 00004 = gender
Var 00005 = mean blood pressure in the first decade
Var 00006 = mean blood pressure in the second decade
Var 00007 = mean blood pressure in the third decade

In the second and third decade an increasing number of patients have been lost. The following time-dependent covariate must be constructed for the analysis of these data (* = sign of multiplication) using the click Transform and click Compute Variable commands:

$(T\_ >=1\&T\_ < 11)*Var\ 5 + (T\_ >=11\&T\_ < 21)*Var\ 6 + (T\_ >=21\&T\_ < 31)*Var\ 7$

This novel predictor variable is entered in the usual way with the commands (Cov = covariate):

Model....time: follow months....status: var 00002....?: define event:1–continue....T_Cov => in box covariates....OK.

The underneath table shows that, indeed, a mean blood pressure after adjustment for difference in decades is a significant predictor of survival at p = 0.040, and with a hazard ratio of 0.936 per mm Hg. In spite of the better blood pressures in the second decade, blood pressure is a significant killer in the overall analysis.

Variables in the Equation

	B	SE	Wald	df	Sig.	Exp(B)
T_COV_	−0.066	0.032	4.238	1	0.040	0.936

13.4 Conclusion

Many predictors of survival change across time, e.g., the effect of smoking, cholesterol, and increased blood pressure in cardiovascular research, and patients' frailty in oncology research.

13.5 Note

More background theoretical and mathematical information is given in Machine Learning in Medicine Part One, Chap. 9, Time-dependent Predictor Modeling, pp 99–111, Springer Heidelberg Germany, 2012, from the same authors.

Chapter 14
Fuzzy Logic for Improved Precision of Dose-Response Data

14.1 General Purpose

Fuzzy logic can handle questions to which the answers may be "yes" at one time and "no" at the other, or may be partially true and untrue. Pharmacodynamic data deal with questions like "does a patient respond to a particular drug dose or not", or "does a drug cause the same effects at the same time in the same subject or not". Such questions are typically of a fuzzy nature, and might, therefore, benefit from an analysis based on fuzzy logic.

14.2 Specific Scientific Question

This chapter is to study whether fuzzy logic can improve the precision of predictive models for pharmacodynamic data.

14.3 Example

Input values	Output values	Fuzzy-modeled output
Induction dosage of thiopental (mg/kg)	Numbers of responders (n)	Numbers of responders (n)
1	4	4
1.5	5	5
2	6	8
2.5	9	10
3	12	12
3.5	17	14
4	17	16
4.5	12	14
5	9	1

We will use as an example the quantal pharmacodynamic effects of different induction dosages of thiopental on numbers of responding subjects. It is usually not possible to know what type of statistical distribution the experiment is likely to

T. J. Cleophas and A. H. Zwinderman, *Machine Learning in Medicine—Cookbook Two*, SpringerBriefs in Statistics, DOI: 10.1007/978-3-319-07413-9_14, © The Author(s) 2014

follow, sometimes Gaussian, sometimes very skewed. A pleasant aspect of fuzzy modeling is that it can be applied with any type of statistical distribution and that it is particularly suitable for uncommon and unexpected non linear relationships.

Quantal response data are often presented in the literature as S-shape dose-cumulative response curves with the dose plotted on a logarithmic scale, where the log transformation has an empirical basis. We will, therefore, use a logarithmic regression model. SPSS Statistical Software is used for analysis.

Command: Analyze...regression...curve estimation...dependent variable: data second column...independent variable: data first column...logarithmic...OK.

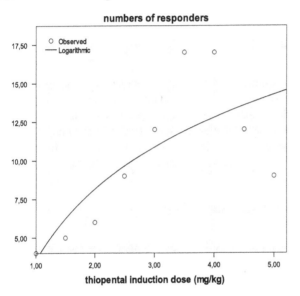

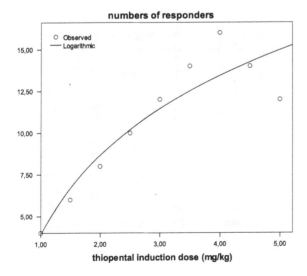

The analysis produces a moderate fit of the data (upper curve) with an r-square value of 0.555 (F-value 8.74, p-value 0.024).

We, subsequently, fuzzy-model the input and output relationships (underneath figure). First of all, we create linguistic rules for the input and output data.

For that purpose we divide the universal space of the input variable into fuzzy memberships with linguistic membership names:

input-*zero, -small, -medium, -big, -superbig.*

Then we do the same for the output variable:

output-*zero, -small, -medium, -big.*

Subsequently, we create linguistic rules.

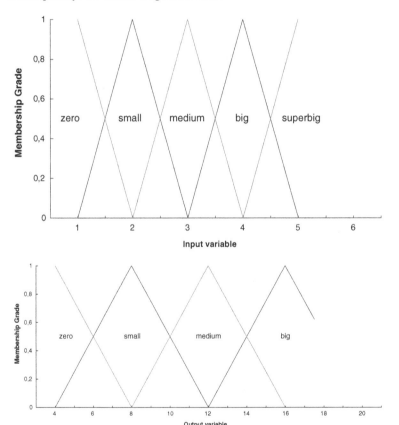

The above figure shows that input-*zero* consists of the values 1 and 1.5.

The value 1 (100 % membership) has 4 as outcome value (100 % membership of output-*zero*).

The value 1.5 (50 % membership) has 5 as outcome value (75 % membership of output-*zero,* 25 % of output-*small*).

The input-*zero* produces 100 % × 100 % + 50 % × 75 % = 137.5 % membership to output-*zero*, and 50 % × 25 % = 12.5 % membership to output-*small*, and so, output-*zero* is the most important output contributor here, and we forget about the small contribution of output-*small*.

Input-*small* is more complex, it consists of the values 1.5, and 2.0, and 2.5.

The value 1.5 (50 % membership) has 5 as outcome value (75 % membership of output-*zero*, 25 % membership of output-*small*).

The value 2.0 (100 % membership) has 6 as outcome value (50 % membership of outcome-*zero*, and 50 % membership of output-*small*).

The value 2.5 (50 % membership) has 9 as outcome value (75 % membership of output-*small* and 25 % of output-*medium*).

The input-*small* produces 50 % × 75 % + 100 % × 50 % = 87.5 % membership to output-*zero*, 50 % × 25 % + 100 % × 50 % + 50 % × 75 % = 100 % membership to output-*small*, and 50 % × 25 % = 12.5 % membership to output-*medium*. And so, the output-*small* is the most important contributor here, and we forget about the other two.

For the other input memberships similar linguistic rules are determined:

Input-*medium* → output-*medium*
Input-*big* → output-*big*
Input-*superbig* → output-*medium*

We are, particularly interested in the modeling capacity of fuzzy logic in order to improve the precision of pharmacodynamic modeling.

The modeled output value of input value 1 is found as follows.

Value 1 is 100 % member of input-*zero*, meaning that according to the above linguistic rules it is also associated with a 100 % membership of output-*zero* corresponding with a value of 4.

Value 1.5 is 50 % member of input-*zero* and 50 % input-*small*. This means it is 50 % associated with the output-*zero* and –*small* corresponding with values of 50 % x (4 + 8) = 6.

For all of the input values modeled output values can be found in this way. Table 19.1 right column shows the results. We perform a logarithmic regression on the fuzzy-modeled outcome data similar to that for the un-modeled output values. The fuzzy-modeled output data provided a much better fit than did the un-modeled output values (lower curve) with an r-square value of 0.852 (F-value = 40.34) as compared to 0.555 (F-value 8.74) for the un-modeled output data.

14.4 Conclusion

Fuzzy logic can handle questions to which the answers may be "yes" at one time and "no" at the other, or may be partially true and untrue. Dose response data deal with questions like "does a patient respond to a particular drug dose or not", or "does a drug cause the same effects at the same time in the same subject or not". Such questions are typically of a fuzzy nature, and might, therefore, benefit from an analysis based on fuzzy logic.

14.5 Note

More background theoretical and mathematical information of analyses using fuzzy logic is given in Machine Learning in Medicine Part One, Chap. 19, pp 241–253, Springer Heidelberg Germany, 2012, from the same authors.

Chapter 15
Automatic Data Mining for the Best Treatment of a Disease (90 Patients)

15.1 General Purpose

SPSS Modeler is a work bench for automatic data mining (current chapter) and data modeling (Chaps. 18, 19). So far it is virtually unused in medicine, and mainly applied by econo-/sociometrists. We will assess whether it can also be used for multiple outcome analysis of clinical data.

15.2 Specific Scientific Question

Patients with sepsis have been given one of three treatments. Various outcome variables are used to assess which one of the treatments performs best.

15.3 Example

In data mining the question "is a treatment a predictor of clinical improvement" is assessed by the question "is the outcome, clinical improvement, a predictor of the chance of having had a treatment". This approach may seem incorrect, but is also used with discriminant analysis, and works fine, because it does not suffer from strong correlations between outcome variables (Machine Learning in Medicine Part One, Chap. 17, Discriminant analysis of supervised data, pp 215–224, Springer Heidelberg, Germany, 2013). In this example, 90 patients with sepsis are treated with three different treatments. Various outcome values are used as predictors of the output treatment.

T. J. Cleophas and A. H. Zwinderman, *Machine Learning in Medicine—Cookbook Two*, SpringerBriefs in Statistics, DOI: 10.1007/978-3-319-07413-9_15, © The Author(s) 2014

Asat	Alat	Ureum	Creat	Crp	Leucos	Treat	Low bp	Death
5.00	29.00	2.40	79.00	18.00	16.00	1.00	1	0
10.00	30.00	2.10	94.00	15.00	15.00	1.00	1	0
8.00	31.00	2.30	79.00	16.00	14.00	1.00	1	0
6.00	16.00	2.70	80.00	17.00	19.00	1.00	1	0
6.00	16.00	2.20	84.00	18.00	20.00	1.00	1	0
5.00	13.00	2.10	78.00	17.00	21.00	1.00	1	0
10.00	16.00	3.10	85.00	20.00	18.00	1.00	1	0
8.00	28.00	8.00	68.00	15.00	18.00	1.00	1	0
7.00	27.00	7.80	74.00	16.00	17.00	1.00	1	0
6.00	26.00	8.40	69.00	18.00	16.00	1.00	1	0
12.00	22.00	2.70	75.00	14.00	19.00	1.00	1	0
21.00	21.00	3.00	70.00	15.00	20.00	1.00	1	0
10.00	20.00	23.00	74.00	15.00	18.00	1.00	1	0
19.00	19.00	2.10	75.00	16.00	16.00	1.00	1	0
8.00	32.00	2.00	85.00	18.00	19.00	1.00	2	0
20.00	11.00	2.90	63.00	18.00	18.00	1.00	1	0
7.00	30.00	6.80	72.00	17.00	18.00	1.00	1	0
1973.00	846.00	73.80	563.00	18.00	38.00	3.00	2	0
1863.00	757.00	41.70	574.00	15.00	34.00	3.00	2	1
1973.00	646.00	38.90	861.00	16.00	38.00	3.00	2	1

Asat = aspartate aminotransferase
Alat = alanine aminotransferase
Creat = creatinine
Crp = c-reactive protein
Treat = treatments 1–3
Low bp = low blood pressure (1 no, 2 slight, 3 severe)
Death = death (0 no, 1 yes)

Only the first 20 patients are above, the entire data file is in extra.springer.com and is entitled "chap15spssmodeler.sav". SPSS Modeler version 14.2 is used for the analysis. Start by opening SPSS Modeler.

15.4   Step 1 Open SPSS Modeler

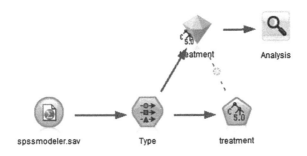

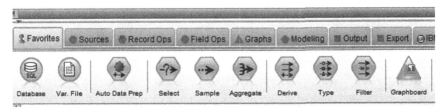

In the palettes at the bottom of the screen full of nodes, look and find the **Statistics File node**, and drag it to the canvas. Double-click on it....Import file: browse and enter the file "chap15spssmodeler.sav"....click OK....in the palette find **Distribution node** and drag to canvas....right-click on the Statistics File node....a Connect symbol comes up....click on the Distribution node....an arrow is displayed....double-click on the Distribution Node....after a second or two the underneath graph with information from the Distribution node is observed.

15.5   Step 2 The Distribution Node

Value /	Proportion	%	Count
1.00		38.89	35
2.00		40.0	36
3.00		21.11	19

It gives the frequency distribution of the three treatments in the 90 patient data file. All of the treatments are substantially present.

Next remove the Distribution node by clicking on it and press delete on the key board of your computer. Continue by dragging the Data audit node to the canvas....perform the connecting manoeuvres as above....double-click it again.

15.6 Step 3 The Data Adit Node

Field	Graph	Measurement	Min	Max	Mean	Std. Dev	Skewness	Unique	Valid
asat		Continuous	5.000	2000.000	360.789	524.433	2.004	--	90
alat		Continuous	11.000	976.000	280.833	318.883	1.036	--	90
ureum		Continuous	2.000	83.000	20.310	19.381	1.338	--	90
creatinine		Continuous	59.000	861.000	272.767	231.551	0.967	--	90
creactiveprotein		Continuous	14.000	131.000	41.667	33.781	1.360	--	90
leucos		Continuous	14.000	42.000	26.822	8.222	0.151	--	90
treatment		Nominal	1.000	3.000	--	--	--	3	90
lowbloodpress...		Nominal	--	--	--	--	--	3	90
death		Nominal	--	--	--	--	--	2	90

The Data audit will be edited. Select "treatment" as target field (field is variable here)....click Run. The information from this node is now given in the form of a Data audit plot, showing that due to the treatment low values are frequently more often observed than the high values. Particularly, the treatments 1 and 2 (light blue and red) are often associated with low values, these are probably the best treatments. Next remove the Data audit node by clicking on it and press delete on the key board of your computer. Continue by dragging the Plot node to the canvas....perform the connecting manoeuvres as above....double-click it again.

15.7 Step 4 The Plot Node

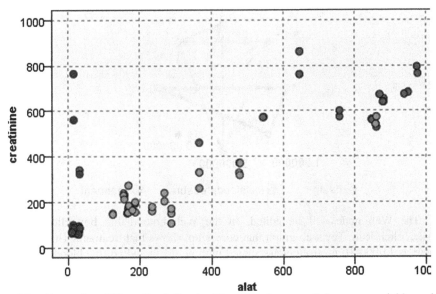

The Plot node will be edited. On the Plot tab select creatinine as y-variable and alat as x-variable, and treatment in the Overlay field at Color....click Run. The information from this node is now given in the form of a scatter plot of patients. This scatter plot of alat versus creatinine values shows that the three treatments are somewhat separately clustered. Treatment 1 (blue) in the left lower part, 2 (green) in the middle, and 3 in the right upper part. Low values means adequate effect of treatment. So treatment 1 (and also some patients with treatment 2) again perform pretty well. Next remove the Plot node by clicking on it and press delete on the key board of your computer. Continue by dragging the Web node to the canvas....perform the connecting manoeuvres as above....double-click it again.

15.8 Step 5 The Web Node

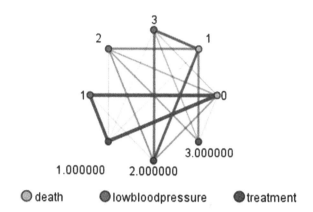

The Web node will be edited. In the Web note dialog box click Select All....click Run. The web graph that comes up, shows that treatment 1 (indicated here as 1.000000) is strongly associated with no death and no low blood pressure (thick line), which is very good. However, the treatments 2 (2.000000) and 3 (3.000000) are strongly associated with death and treatment 2 (2.000000) is also associated with the severest form of low blood pressure. Next remove the Web node by clicking on it and press delete on the key board of your computer. Continue by dragging both the Type and C5.0 nodes to the canvas....perform the connecting manoeuvres respectively as indicated in the first graph of this chapter....double-click it again....a gold nugget is placed as shown above....click the gold nugget.

15.9 Step 6 The Type and C5.0 Nodes

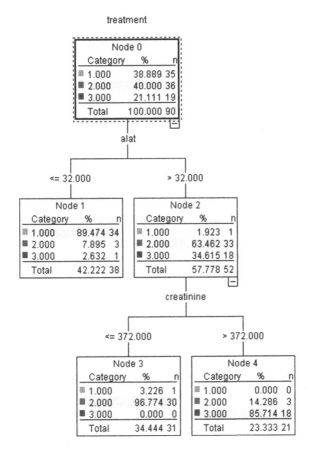

The output sheets give various interactive graphs and tables. One of them is the above C5.0 decision tree. C5.0 decision trees are an improved version of the traditional Quinlan decision trees with less, but more-relevant information.

The C5.0 classifier underscores the previous findings. The variable alat is the best classifier of the treatments with alat < 32 over 89 % of the patients having had treatment 1, and with alat > 32 over 63 % of the patients having had treatment 2. Furthermore, in the high alat class patients with a creatinine over 372 around 86 % has treatment 3. And so all in all, the treatment 1 would seem the best treatment and treatment 3 the worst one.

15.10 Step 7 The Output Node

⊟ Results for output field treatment
  ⊟ Comparing $C-treatment with treatment

Correct	82	91,11%
Wrong	8	8,89%
Total	90	

In order to assess the accuracy of the C5.0 classifier output an Output node is attached to the gold nugget. Find Output node and drag it to the canvas....perform connecting manoeuvres with the gold nugget....double-click the Output node again....click Run. The output sheet shows an accuracy (true positives and true negatives) of 91.11 %, which is pretty good.

15.11 Conclusion

SPSS Modeler can be adequately used for multiple outcomes analysis of clinical data. Finding the most appropriate treatment for a disease might be one of the goals of this kind of research.

15.12 Note

SPSS Modeler is a software program entirely distinct from SPSS statistical software, though it uses most if not all of the calculus methods of it. It is a standard software package particularly used by market analysts, but as shown can, perfectly, well be applied for exploratory purposes in medical research.

Chapter 16
Pareto Charts for Identifying the Main Factors of Multifactorial Outcomes

16.1 General Purpose

In 1906 the Italian economist Pareto observed that 20 % of the Italian population possessed 80 % of the land, and, looking at other countries, virtually the same seemed to be true. The Pareto principle is currently used to identify the main factors of multifactorial outcomes. Pareto charts is available in SPSS, and this chapter is to assess whether it is useful, not only in marketing science, but also in medicine.

16.2 Primary Scientific Question

To assess whether pareto charts can be applied to identify in a study of hospital admissions the main causes of iatrogenic admissions.

16.3 Example

2000 subsequent admissions to a general hospital in the Netherlands were classified.

Indications for admission	Numbers	(%)	Confidence intervals (95 %)
1. Cardiac condition and hypertension	810	40.5	38.0–42.1
2. Gastrointestinal condition	254	12.7	11.9–14.2
3. Infectious disease	200	10.0	9.2–12.0
4. Pulmonary disease	137	6.9	6.5–7.7

(continued)

(continued)

Indications for admission	Numbers	(%)	Confidence intervals (95 %)
5. Hematological condition	109	5.5	4.0–6.2
6. Malignancy	74	3.7	2.7–4.9
7. Mental disease	54	2.7	1.9–3.8
8. Endocrine condition	49	2.5	1.7–3.5
9. Bleedings with acetyl salicyl/NSAIDS	47	2.4	1.6–3.4
10. Other	41	2.1	1.4–3.1
11. Unintentional overdose	31	1.6	1.0–2.5
12. Bleeding with acenocoumarol/dalteparin	28	1.4	0.8–2.2
13. Fever after chemotherapy	26	1.3	0.7–2.1
14. Electrolyte disturbance	26	1.3	0.7–2.1
15. Dehydration	23	1.2	0.7–2.0
16. Other problems after chemotherapy	20	1.0	0.5–1.8
17. Allergic reaction	17	0.9	0.4–1.7
18. Renal disease	16	0.8	0.3–1.5
19. Pain syndrome	8	0.4	0.1–1.0
20. Hypotension	8	0.4	0.1–1.0
21. Neurological disease	7	0.4	0.1–1.0
22. Vascular disease	6	0.3	0.06–0.7
23. Rheumatoid arthritis/arthrosis/osteoporosis	6	0.3	0.06–0.7
24. Dermatological condition	3	0.2	0.02–0.7
	2000	100	

NSAIDS = non-steroidal anti-inflammatory drugs

The data file is in extras.springer.com and is entitled "Chap. 16pareto-charts.sav". Open it.

Command:

Analyze....Quality Control....Pareto Charts....click Simple....mark Value of individual cases....click Define....Values: enter "alladmissions"....mark Variable: enter "diagnosisgroups"....click OK.

The underneath graph shows that over 50 % of the admissions is in the first two diagnosis groups. A general rule as postulated by Pareto says: when analyzing observational studies with multifactorial effects, usually less than 20 % of the factors determines over 80 % of the effect. This postulate seems to be true in this example. The graph shows that the first 5 diagnosis groups out of 21 % determine around 80 % of the effect (admission). When launching a program to reduce hospital admissions in general, it would make sense to prioritize these 5 diagnosis groups, and to neglect the other diagnosis groups.

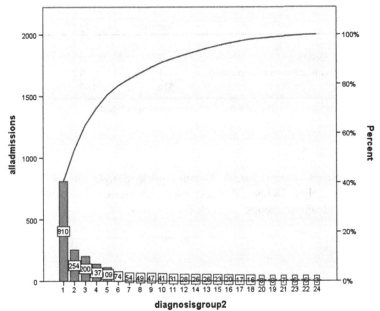

diagnosisgroup2

In order to find out how diagnosis groups contributed to the numbers of iatrogenic admissions, a pareto chart was constructed. The data are underneath, and are the variables 4 and 5 in "Chap16paretocharts.sav".

	Numbers	(%)	95 % CIs
1. Cardiac condition and hypertension	202	35.1	31.1–38.9
2. Gastrointestinal condition	89	15.5	12.2–18.1
3. Bleedings with acetyl salicyl/NSAIDS	46	8.0	5.9–10.4
4. Infectious disease	31	5.4	3.6–7.4
5. Bleeding with acenocoumarol/dalteparin	28	4.9	3.1–6.8
6. Fever after chemotherapy	26	4.5	2.9–6.4
7. Hematological condition	24	4.2	2.7–6.1
8. Other problems after chemotherapy	20	3.5	2.1–5.3
9. Endocrine condition	19	3.3	2.0–5.1
10. Dehydration	18	3.1	1.9–4.9
11. Electrolyte disturbance	14	2.4	1.3–3.8
12. Pulmonary disease	9	1.6	0.8–3.0
13. Allergic reaction	8	1.4	0.6–2.8
14. Hypotension not due to antihypertensives	8	1.4	0.6–2.8
15. Other	7	1.2	0.5–2.4
16. Unintentional overdose	6	1.0	0.4–2.1
17. Malignancy	6	1.0	0.4–2.1
18. Neurological disease	4	0.7	0.2–1.7
19. Mental disease	4	0.7	0.2–1.7
20. Renal disease	2	0.3	0.04–1.2

(continued)

(continued)

	Numbers	(%)	95 % CIs
21. Vascular disease	2	0.3	0.04–1.2
22. Dermatological condition	2	0.3	0.04–1.2
23. Rheumatoid arthritis/arthrosis/osteoporosis	1	0.2	0.0–0.9
Total	576	100	

NSAIDS = non-steroidal anti-inflammatory drugs; ns = not significant

Command:
Analyze....Quality Control....Pareto Charts....click Simple....mark Value of individual cases....click Define....Values: enter "iatrogenicadmissions"....mark Variable: enter "diagnosisgroups"....click OK.

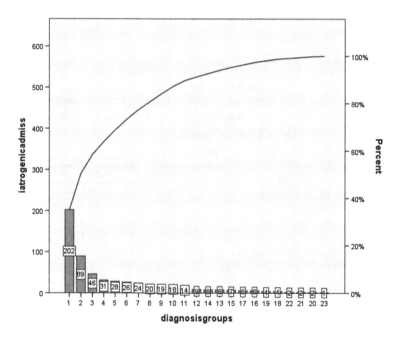

The above pareto chart has a breakpoint at 50 %. Generally, a breakpoint is observed at around 50 % of the effect with around 10 % of the factors before the breakpoint. The breakpoint would be helpful for setting priorities, when addressing the problem of iatrogenic admissions. The diagnosis groups, cardiac condition and gastrointestinal condition, cause over 50 % of all of the iatrogenic admissions.

In order to find which medicines were responsible for the iatrogenic admissions, again a pareto chart was constructed. The variables 1 and 2 of the data file " Chap. 16 paretocharts.sav" will be used.

Command:
Analyzed....Quality Control....Pareto Charts....click Simple....mark Value of individual cases....click Define....Values: enter "iatrogenicad"....mark Variable: enter "medicinecat"....click OK.

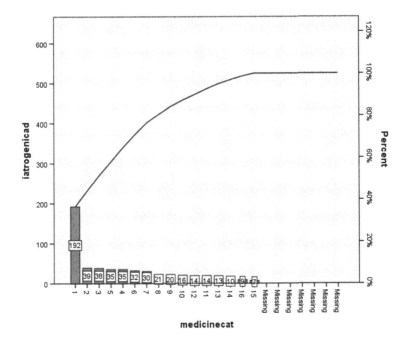

No breakpoint is observed, but the first two medicine categories were responsible for 50 % of the entire number of iatrogenic admissions. We can conclude, that over 50 % of the iatrogenic admissions were in two diagnosis groups, and over 50 % of the medicines responsible were also in two main medicine categories.

16.4 Conclusion

Pareto charts are useful for identifying the main factors of multifactorial outcomes, not only in marketing science but also in medicine.

16.5 Note

In addition to flow charts, scattergrams, histograms, control charts, cause effects diagrams, and checklists, pareto charts are basic graphical tools of data analysis. All of them require little training in statistics.

Chapter 17
Radial Basis Neural Networks
for Multidimensional Gaussian Data
(90 Persons)

17.1 General Purpose

Radial basis functions may better than multilayer neural network (Machine Learning in Medicine Cookbook One, Chap. 13, Neural networks for assessing relationships that are typically nonlinear, pp 81–83, Springer Heidelberg Germany, 2014, from the same authors) predict medical data, because it uses a Gaussian activation function, but it is rarely used. This chapter is to assess its performance in clinical research.

17.2 Specific Scientific Question

Body surface area is an indicator for metabolic body mass, and is used for adjusting oxygen, CO_2 transport parameters, blood volumes, urine creatinine clearance, protein/creatinine ratios and other parameters. Can a radial basis neural network be applied to accurately predict the body surface from gender, age, weight and height?

17.3 Example

The body surfaces of 90 persons were calculated using direct photometric measurements. These previously measured outcome data will be used as the socalled learning sample, and the computer will be commanded to teach itself making predictions about the body surface from the predictor variables gender, age, weight and height. The first 20 patients are underneath. The entire data file is in "chap17 radialbasisnn".

T. J. Cleophas and A. H. Zwinderman, *Machine Learning in Medicine—Cookbook Two*, SpringerBriefs in Statistics, DOI: 10.1007/978-3-319-07413-9_17, © The Author(s) 2014

1.00	13.00	30.50	138.50	10072.90
0.00	5.00	15.00	101.00	6189.00
0.00	0.00	2.50	51.50	1906.20
1.00	11.00	30.00	141.00	10290.60
1.00	15.00	40.50	154.00	13221.60
0.00	11.00	27.00	136.00	9654.50
0.00	5.00	15.00	106.00	6768.20
1.00	5.00	15.00	103.00	6194.10
1.00	3.00	13.50	96.00	5830.20
0.00	13.00	36.00	150.00	11759.00
0.00	3.00	12.00	92.00	5299.40
1.00	0.00	2.50	51.00	2094.50
0.00	7.00	19.00	121.00	7490.80
1.00	13.00	28.00	130.50	9521.70
1.00	0.00	3.00	54.00	2446.20
0.00	0.00	3.00	51.00	1632.50
0.00	7.00	21.00	123.00	7958.80
1.00	11.00	31.00	139.00	10580.80
1.00	7.00	24.50	122.50	8756.10
1.00	11.00	26.00	133.00	9573.00

Var 1 gender
Var 2 age
Var 3 weight (kg)
Var 4 height (m)
Var 5 body surface measured (cm^2)

17.4 The Computer Teaches Itself to Make Predictions

The SPSS module Neural Networks is used for training and outcome prediction. It uses XML (exTended Markup Language) files to store the neural network. Start by opening the data file.

Command:

click Transform….click Random Number Generators….click Set Starting Point….click Fixed Value (2000000)….click OK….click Analyze…. Neural Networks….Radial Basis Function….Dependent Variables: enter Body surface measured….Factors: enter gender, age, weight, and height….Partitions: Training 7….Test 3….Holdout 0….click Output: mark Description….Diagram…. Model summary….Predicted by observed chart….Case processing summary ….click Save: mark Save predicted value of category for each dependent variable….automatically generate unique names….click Export….mark Export synaptic weights estimates to XML file….click Browse….File Name: enter "exportradialbasisnn" and save in the appropriate folder of your computer….click OK.

The output warns that in the testing sample some cases have been excluded from analysis, because of values not occurring in the training sample. Minimizing the output sheets shows the data file with predicted values. They are pretty much the same as the measured body surface values. We will use linear regression to estimate the association between the two.

Command:

Analyze....Regresssion....Linear....Dependent: bodysurface ....Independent: RBF_PredictedValue....OK.

The output sheets show that the r-value is 0.931, $p < 0.0001$. The saved XML file will now be used to compute the body surface in six individual patients.

Gender	Age	Weight	Height
1.00	9.00	29.00	138.00
1.00	1.00	8.00	76.00
0.00	15.00	42.00	165.00
1.00	15.00	40.00	151.00
1.00	1.00	9.00	80.00
1.00	7.00	22.00	123.00

Gender
Age (years)
Weight (kg)
Height (m)

Enter the above data in a new SPSS data file.

Command:

Utilities....click Scoring Wizard....click Browse....click Select....Folder: enter the exportradialbasisnn.xml file....click Select....in Scoring Wizard click Next....click Use value substitution....click Next....click Finish.

The underneath data file now gives the body surfaces computed by the neural network with the help of the XML file.

Gender	Age	Weight	Height	Predicted body surface
1.00	9.00	29.00	138.00	9219.71
1.00	1.00	8.00	76.00	5307.81
0.00	15.00	42.00	165.00	13520.13
1.00	15.00	40.00	151.00	13300.79
1.00	1.00	9.00	80.00	5170.13
1.00	7.00	22.00	123.00	8460.05

Gender
Age (years)
Weight (kg)
Height (m)
Predicted body surface (cm^2)

17.5 Conclusion

Radial basis neural networks can be readily trained to provide accurate body surface values of individual patients.

17.6 Note

More background, theoretical and mathematical information of neural networks is available in Machine Learning in Medicine Part One, Chaps. 12 and 13, entitled "Artificial intelligence, multilayer perceptron" and "Artificial intelligence, radial basis functions", pp 145–156 and 157–166, Springer Heidelberg Germany 2013.

Chapter 18
Automatic Modeling of Drug Efficacy Prediction (250 Patients)

18.1 General Purpose

SPSS Modeler is a work bench for automatic data mining (Chap. 15) and modeling (Chaps. 18, 19). So far it is virtually unused in medicine, and mainly applied by econo-/sociometrists. Automatic modeling of continuous outcomes computes the ensembled result of a number of best fit models for a particular data set, and provides better sensitivity than the separate models do. This chapter is to demonstrate its performance with drug efficacy prediction.

18.2 Specific Scientific Question

The expression of a cluster of genes can be used as a functional unit to predict the efficacy of cytostatic treatment. Can ensembled modeling with three best fit statistical models provide better precision than the separate analysis with single statistical models does.

18.3 Example

A 250 patients' data file includes 28 variables consistent of patients' gene expression levels and their drug efficacy scores. Only the first 12 patients are shown underneath. The entire data file is in extras.springer.com, and is entitled "chap18ensembledmodelcontinuous". All of the variables were standardized by scoring them on 11 points linear scales. The following genes were highly expressed: the genes 1–4, 16–19, and 24–27.

T. J. Cleophas and A. H. Zwinderman, *Machine Learning in Medicine—Cookbook Two*, SpringerBriefs in Statistics, DOI: 10.1007/978-3-319-07413-9_18, © The Author(s) 2014

G1	G2	G3	G4	G16	G17	G18	G19	G24	G25	G26	G27	O
8.00	8.00	9.00	5.00	7.00	10.00	5.00	6.00	9.00	9.00	6.00	6.00	7.00
9.00	9.00	10.00	9.00	8.00	8.00	7.00	8.00	8.00	9.00	8.00	8.00	7.00
9.00	8.00	8.00	8.00	8.00	9.00	7.00	8.00	9.00	8.00	9.00	9.00	8.00
8.00	9.00	8.00	9.00	6.00	7.00	6.00	4.00	6.00	6.00	5.00	5.00	7.00
10.00	10.00	8.00	10.00	9.00	10.00	10.00	8.00	8.00	9.00	9.00	9.00	8.00
7.00	8.00	8.00	8.00	8.00	7.00	6.00	5.00	7.00	8.00	8.00	7.00	6.00
5.00	5.00	5.00	5.00	5.00	6.00	4.00	5.00	5.00	6.00	6.00	5.00	5.00
9.00	9.00	9.00	9.00	8.00	8.00	8.00	8.00	9.00	8.00	3.00	8.00	8.00
9.00	8.00	9.00	8.00	9.00	8.00	7.00	7.00	7.00	7.00	5.00	8.00	7.00
10.00	10.00	10.00	10.00	10.00	10.00	10.00	10.00	10.00	8.00	8.00	10.00	10.00
2.00	2.00	8.00	5.00	7.00	8.00	8.00	8.00	9.00	3.00	9.00	8.00	7.00
7.00	8.00	8.00	7.00	8.00	6.00	6.00	7.00	8.00	8.00	8.00	7.00	7.00

G = gene (gene expression levels), O = outcome(score)

18.4 Step 1: Open SPSS Modeler (14.2)

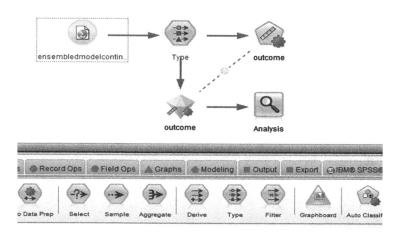

18.5 Step 2: The Statistics File Node

The canvas is, initially, blank, and above a screen view is of the final "completed ensemble" model, otherwise called stream of nodes, which we are going to build. First, in the palettes at the bottom of the screen full of nodes, look and find the **Statistics File node**, and drag it to the canvas. Double-click on it....Import file: browse and enter the file "chap18ensembledmodelcontinuous" ....click OK. The graph below shows that the data file is open for analysis.

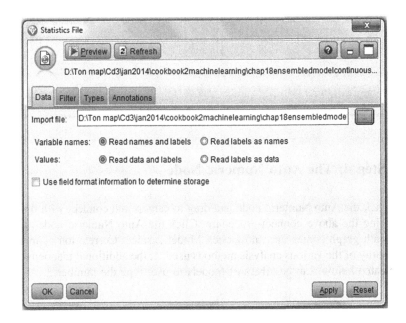

18.6 Step 3: The Type Node

In the palette at the bottom of screen find Type node and drag to the canvas....right-click on the Statistics File node....a Connect symbol comes up....click on the Type node....an arrow is displayed....double-click on the Type Node....after a second or two the underneath graph with information from the Type node is observed. Type nodes are used to access the properties of the variables (often called fields here) like type, role, unit etc. in the data file. As shown below, the variables are appropriately set: 14 predictor variables, 1 outcome (=target) variable, all of them continuous.

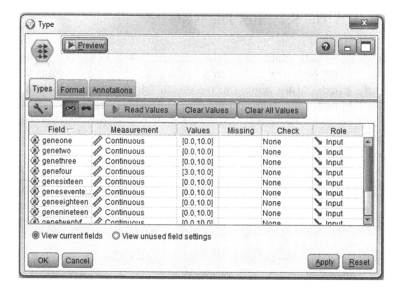

18.7 Step 4: The Auto Numeric Node

Now, click the Auto Numeric node and drag to canvas and connect with the Type node using the above connect-procedure. Click the Auto Numeric node, and the underneath graph comes up....now click Model....select Correlation as metric to rank quality of the various analysis methods used.... the additional manoeuvres are as indicated below....in Numbers of models to use: type the number 3.

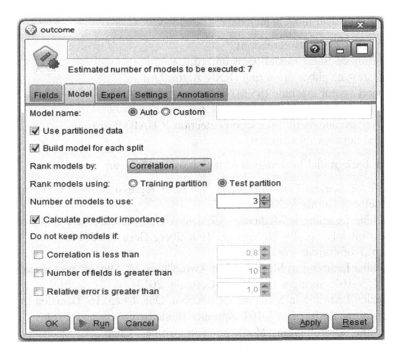

18.8 Step 5: The Expert Node

Then click the Expert tab. It is shown below. Out of 7 statistical models the three best fit ones are used by SPSS Modeler for the ensembled model.

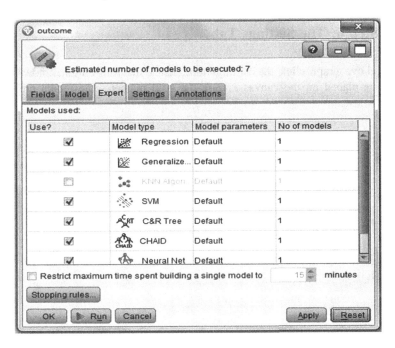

The 7 statistical models include:

1. Linear regression (Regression)
2. Generalized linear model (Generalized....)
3. K nearest neighbor clustering (KNN Algorithm)
4. Support vector machine (SVM)
5. Classification and regression tree (C&R Tree)
6. Chi square automatic interaction detection (CHAID Tree)
7. Neural network (Neural Net)

More background information of the above methods are available at

1. SPSS for Starters Part One, Chap. 5, Linear regression, pp. 15–18, Springer Heidelberg Germany 2010,
2. Machine Learning in Medicine—Cookbook One, Chaps. 5 and 6, Generalized linear models, pp. 29–41, Springer Heidelberg Germany 2014,
3. Chap. 1 of current work,
4. Machine Learning in Medicine Part Two, Chap. 15, Support vector machines, pp. 155–161, Springer Heidelberg Germany 2013,
5. Machine Learning in Medicine—Cookbook One, Chap. 16, Decision trees for decision analysis, pp. 97–104, Springer Heidelberg Germany 2014,
6. Machine Learning in Medicine Part Three, Chap. 14, Decision trees, pp. 137–150, Springer Heidelberg Germany 2013,
7. Machine Learning in Medicine Part One, Chap. 12, Artificial intelligence, multilayer perceptron modeling, pp. 145–154, Springer Heidelberg Germany 2013.

All of the seven above references are from the same authors as the current work.

18.9 Step 6: The Settings Tab

In the above graph click the Settings tab....click the Run button....now a gold nugget is placed on the canvas....click the gold nugget....the model created is shown below.

Use?	Graph	Model	Build Time (mins)	Correlation	No. Fields Used	Relative Error
☑		CHAID 1	< 1	0,854	8	0,271
☑		SVM 1	< 1	0,836	12	0,304
☑		Regressi...	< 1	0,821	12	0,326

The correlation coefficients of the three best models are over 0.8, and, thus, pretty good. We will now perform the ensembled procedure.

18.10 Step 7: The Analysis Node

Find in the palettes below the screen the Analysis node and drag it to the canvas. With the above connect procedure connect it with the gold nugget....click the Analysis node.

Comparing $XR-outcome with outcome

Minimum Error	-2,878
Maximum Error	3,863
Mean Error	-0,014
Mean Absolute Error	0,77
Standard Deviation	1,016
Linear Correlation	0,859
Occurrences	250

The above table is shown and gives the statistics of the ensembled model created. The ensembled outcome is the average score of the scores from the three best fit statistical models. Adjustment for multiple testing and for variance stabilization with Fisher transformation is automatically carried out. The ensembled outcome (named the $XR-outcome) is compared with the outcomes of the three best fit statistical models, namely, CHAID (chi square automatic interaction detector), SVM (support vector machine), and Regression (linear regression). The ensembled correlation coefficient is larger (0.859) than the correlation coefficients from the three best fit models (0.854, 0.836, 0.821), and so ensembled procedures make sense, because they can provide increased precision in the analysis. The ensembled model can now be stored as an SPSS Modeler Stream file for future use in the appropriate folder of your computer. For the readers' convenience it is in extras.springer.com, and it is entitled "ensembledmodelcontinuous".

18.11 Conclusion

In the example given in this chapter, the ensembled correlation coefficient is larger (0.859) than the correlation coefficients from the three best fit models (0.854, 0.836, 0.821), and, so, ensembled procedures do make sense, because they can provide increased precision in the analysis.

18.12 Note

SPSS Modeler is a software program entirely distinct from SPSS statistical software, though it uses most if not all of the calculus methods of it. It is a standard software package particularly used by market analysts, but, as shown, can, perfectly, well be applied for exploratory purposes in medical research.

Chapter 19
Automatic Modeling for Clinical Event Prediction (200 Patients)

19.1 General Purpose

SPSS Modeler is a work bench for automatic data mining and modeling (Chap. 15) and modeling (Chaps. 18 and 19). So far it is virtually unused in medicine, and mainly applied by econo-/sociometrists. Automatic modeling of binary outcomes computes the ensembled result of a number of best fit models for a particular data set, and provides better sensitivity than the separate models do. This chapter is to demonstrate its performance with clinical event prediction.

19.2 Specific Scientific Question

Multiple laboratory values can predict events like health, death, morbidities etc. Can ensembled modeling with four best fit statistical models provide better precision than the separate analysis with single statistical models does.

19.3 Example

A 200 patients' data file includes 11 variables consistent of patients' laboratory values and their subsequent outcome (death or alive). Only the first 12 patients are shown underneath. The entire data file is in extras.springer.com, and is entitled "chap19ensembledmodelbinary".

Death	ggt	asat	alat	bili	ureum	creat	c-clear	esr	crp	leucos
0.00	20.00	23.00	34.00	2.00	3.40	89.00	−111.00	2.00	2.00	5.00
0.00	14.00	21.00	33.00	3.00	2.00	67.00	−112.00	7.00	3.00	6.00

(continued)

T. J. Cleophas and A. H. Zwinderman, *Machine Learning in Medicine—Cookbook Two*, SpringerBriefs in Statistics, DOI: 10.1007/978-3-319-07413-9_19, © The Author(s) 2014

(continued)

Death	ggt	asat	alat	bili	ureum	creat	c-clear	esr	crp	leucos
0.00	30.00	35.00	32.00	4.00	5.60	58.00	−116.00	8.00	4.00	4.00
0.00	35.00	34.00	40.00	4.00	6.00	76.00	−110.00	6.00	5.00	7.00
0.00	23.00	33.00	22.00	4.00	6.10	95.00	−120.00	9.00	6.00	6.00
0.00	26.00	31.00	24.00	3.00	5.40	78.00	−132.00	8.00	4.00	8.00
0.00	15.00	29.00	26.00	2.00	5.30	47.00	−120.00	12.00	5.00	5.00
0.00	13.00	26.00	24.00	1.00	6.30	65.00	−132.00	13.00	6.00	6.00
0.00	26.00	27.00	27.00	4.00	6.00	97.00	−112.00	14.00	6.00	7.00
0.00	34.00	25.00	13.00	3.00	4.00	67.00	−125.00	15.00	7.00	6.00
0.00	32.00	26.00	24.00	3.00	3.60	58.00	−110.00	13.00	8.00	6.00
0.00	21.00	13.00	15.00	3.00	3.60	69.00	−102.00	12.00	2.00	4.00

death = death yes no (0 = no)
ggt = gamma glutamyl transferase (u/l)
asat = aspartate aminotransferase (u/l)
alat = alanine aminotransferase (u/l)
bili = bilirubine (micromol/l)
ureum = ureum (mmol/l)
creat = creatinine (mmicromol/l)
c-clear = creatinine clearance (ml/min)
esr = erythrocyte sedimentation rate (mm)
crp = c-reactive protein (mg/l)
leucos = leucocyte count ($\cdot 10^9$ /l)

19.4 Step 1: Open SPSS Modeler (14.2)

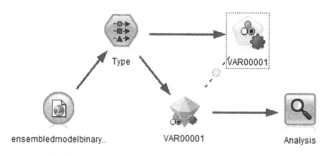

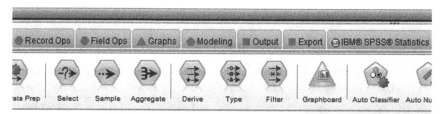

19.5   Step 2: The Statistics File Node

The canvas is, initially, blank, and above is given a screen view of the completed ensembled model, otherwise called stream of nodes, which we are going to build. First, in the palettes at the bottom of the screen full of nodes, look and find the **Statistics File node**, and drag it to the canvas, pressing the mouse left side. Double-click on this node....Import file: browse and enter the file "chap19en-sembledmodelbinary" ....click OK. The graph below shows, that the data file is open for analysis.

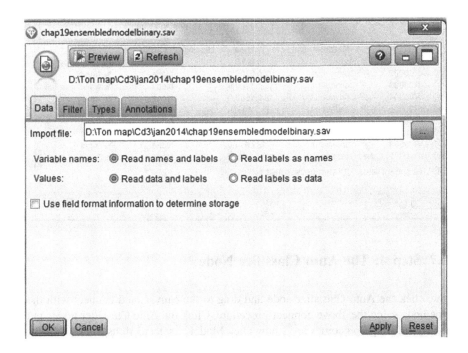

19.6   Step 3: The Type Node

In the palette at the bottom of screen find Type node and drag to the can-vas....right-click on the Statistics File node....a Connect symbol comes up....click on the Type node....an arrow is displayed....double-click on the Type Node....-after a second or two the underneath graph with information from the Type node is observed. Type nodes are used to access the properties of the variables (often called fields here) like type, role, unit etc. in the data file. As shown below, 10 predictor variables (all of them continuous) are appropriately set. However, VAR 00001 (death) is the outcome (= target) variable, and is binary. Click in the row of variable VAR00001 on the measurement column and replace "Continuous" with "Flag". Click Apply and OK. The underneath figure is removed and the canvas is displayed again.

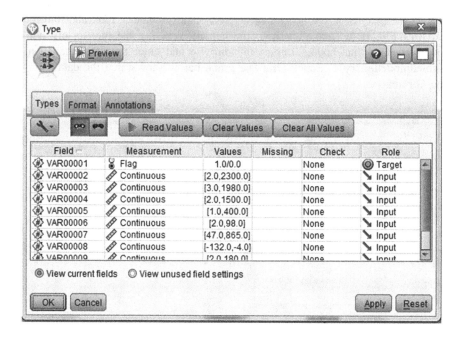

19.7 Step 4: The Auto Classifier Node

Now, click the Auto Classifier node and drag to the canvas, and connect with the Type node using the above connect-procedure. Click the Auto Classifier node, and the underneath graph comes up....now click Model....select Lift as Rank model of the various analysis models used.... the additional manoeuvres are as indicated below....in Numbers of models to use: type the number 4.

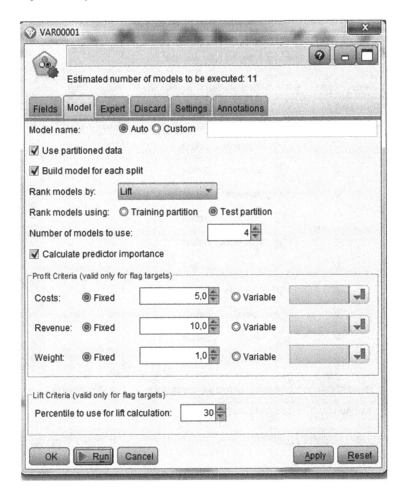

19.8 Step 5: The Expert Tab

Then click the Expert tab. It is shown below. Out of 11 statistical models the four
best fit ones are selected by SPSS Modeler for constructing an ensembled model.

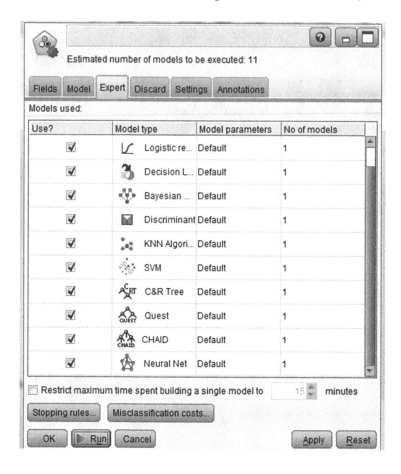

The 11 statistical analysis methods for a flag target (= binary outcome) include:

1. C5.0 decision tree (C5.0)
2. Logistic regression (Logist r...)
3. Decision list (Decision....)
4. Bayesian network (Bayesian....)
5. Discriminant analysis (Discriminant)
6. K nearest neighbors algorithm (KNN Alg...)
7. Support vector machine (SVM)
8. Classification and regression tree (C&R Tree)
9. Quest decision tree (Quest Tr....)
10. Chi square automatic interaction detection (CHAID Tree)
11. Neural network (Neural Net)

More background information of the above methods are available at

1. Chap. 15 of current work, Automatic data mining for the best treatment of a disease,
2. SPSS for Starters Part One, Chap. 11, Logistic regression, pp 39–42, Springer Heidelberg Germany 2010
3. Decision list models identify high and low performing segments in a data file,
4. Machine Learning in Medicine Part Two, Chap. 16, s, pp 163–170, Springer Heidelberg Germany, 2013,
5. Machine Learning in Medicine Part One, Chap. 17, Discriminant analysis for supervised data, pp 215–224, Springer Heidelberg Germany 2013,
6. Chap. 1 of current work, Nearest neighbors for classifying new medicines,
7. Machine Learning in Medicine Part Two, Chap. 15, Support vector machines, pp 155–161, Springer Heidelberg Germany, 2013,
8. Machine Learning in Medicine—Cookbook One, Chap. 16, Decision trees for decision analysis, pp 97–104, Springer Heidelberg Germany 2014,
9. Quick Unbiased Efficient Statistical Trees (QUEST) are improved Decision trees for binary outcomes,
10. Machine Learning in Medicine Part Three, Chap. 14, Decision trees, pp 137–150, Springer Heidelberg Germany 2013,
11. Machine Learning in Medicine Part One, Chap. 12, Artificial intelligence, multilayer perceptron modeling, pp 145–154, Springer Heidelberg Germany 2013.

All of the above references are from the same authors as the current work.

19.9 Step 6: The Settings Tab

In the above graph click the Settings tab....click the Run button....now a gold nugget is placed on the canvas....click the gold nugget....the model created is shown below.

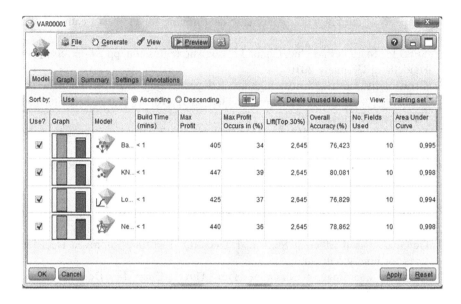

The overall accuracies (%) of the four best fit models are between 76.4 and 80.1, and are, thus, pretty good. We will now perform the ensembled procedure.

19.10 Step 7: The Analysis Node

Find in the palettes at the bottom of the screen the Analysis node and drag it to the canvas. With above connect procedure connect it with the gold nugget....click the Analysis node.

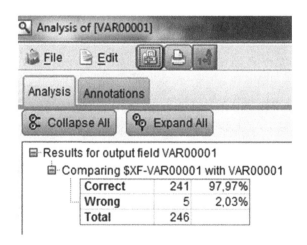

The above table is shown and gives the statistics of the ensembled model created. The ensembled outcome is the Average accuracy of the accuracies from the four best fit statistical models. In order to prevent overstated certainty due to overfitting , bootstrap aggregating ("bagging") is used. The ensembled outcome (named the $XR-outcome) is compared with the outcomes of the four best fit statistical models, namely, Bayesian network, k Nearest Neighbor clustering, Logistic regression, and Neural network. The ensembled accuracy (97.97 %) is much larger than the accuracies of the four best fit models (76.423, 80,081, 76,829, and 78,862 %), and, so, ensembled procedures make sense, because they provide increased precision in the analysis. The computed ensembled model can now be stored in your computer in the form of an SPSS Modeler Stream file for future use. For the readers' convenience it is in extras.springer.com, and entitled "ensembledmodelbinary".

19.11 Conclusion

In the example given in this chapter, the ensembled accuracy is larger (97,97 %) than the accuracies from the four best fit models (76.423, 80,081, 76,829, and 78,862 %), and so ensembled procedures make sense, because they can provide increased precision in the analysis.

19.12 Note

SPSS Modeler is a software program entirely distinct from SPSS statistical software, though it uses most if not all of the calculus methods of it. It is a standard software package particularly used by market analysts, but, as shown, can perfectly well be applied for exploratory purposes in medical research.

Chapter 20
Automatic Newton Modeling in Clinical Pharmacology (15 Alfentanil Dosages, 15 Quinidine Time-Concentration Relationships)

20.1 General Purpose

Traditional regression analysis selects a mathematical function, and, then, uses the data to find the best fit parameters. For example, the parameters a and b for a linear regression function with the equation $y = a + bx$ have to be calculated according to

$$b = \text{regression coefficient} = \frac{\sum (x - \bar{x})(y - \bar{y})}{\sum (x - \bar{x})^2}.$$

$$a = \text{intercept } \bar{y} - b\bar{x}$$

With a quadratic function, $y = a + b_1x + b_2x^2$ (and other functions) the calculations are similar, but more complex. Newton's method works differently [1]. Instead of selecting a mathematical function and using the data for finding the best fit parameter-values, it uses arbitrary parameter-values for a, b_1, b_2, and, then, iteratively measures the distance between the data and the modeled curve until the shortest distance is obtained. Calculations are much more easy than those of traditional regression analysis, making the method, particularly, interesting for comparing multiple functions to one data set. Newton's method is mainly used for computer solutions of engineering problems, but is little used in clinical research. This chapter is to assess whether it is also suitable for the latter purpose.

20.2 Specific Scientific Question

Can Newton's methods provide appropriate mathematical functions for dose-effectiveness and time-concentration studies?

T. J. Cleophas and A. H. Zwinderman, *Machine Learning in Medicine—Cookbook Two*, SpringerBriefs in Statistics, DOI: 10.1007/978-3-319-07413-9_20, © The Author(s) 2014

20.3 Examples

20.3.1 Dose-Effectiveness Study

Alfentanil dose x-axis mg/m^2	Effectiveness y-axis (1-pain scale)
0.10	0.1701
0.20	0.2009
0.30	0.2709
0.40	0.2648
0.50	0.3013
0.60	0.4278
0.70	0.3466
0.80	0.2663
0.90	0.3201
1.00	0.4140
1.10	0.3677
1.20	0.3476
1.30	0.3656
1.40	0.3879
1.50	0.3649

The above table gives the data of a dose-effectiveness study. Newton's algorithm is performed. We will the online Nonlinear Regression Calculator of Xuru's website (This website is made available by Xuru, the world largest business network based in Auckland CA, USA. We simply copy or paste the data of the above table into the spreadsheet given be the website, then click "allow comma as decimal separator" and click "calculate". Alternatively the SPSS file available at extras.springer.com entitled "chap20newtonmethod" can be opened if SPSS is installed in your computer and the copy and paste commands are similarly given.

Since Newton's method can be applied to (almost) any function, most computer programs fit a given dataset to over 100 functions including Gaussians, sigmoids, ratios, sinusoids etc. For the data given 18 significantly ($P < 0.05$) fitting nonlinear functions were found, the first 6 of them are shown underneath.

	Non-linear function	Residual sum of squares	P value
1.	$y = 0.42\,x/(x + 0.17)$	0.023	0.003
2.	$y = -1/(38.4\,x + 1)^{0.12} + 1$	0.024	0.003
3.	$y = 0.08\,\ln x + 0.36$	0.025	0.004
4.	$y = 0.40\,e^{-0.11/x}$	0.025	0.004
5.	$y = 0.36\,x^{0.26}$	0.027	0.004
6.	$y = -0.024/x + 0.37$	0.029	0.005

The first one gives the best fit. Its measure of certainty, given as residual sum of squares, is 0.023. It is the function of a hyperbola:

$$y = 0.42\,x/(x + 0.17).$$

This is convenient, because, dose-effectiveness curves are, often, successfully assessed with hyperbolas mimicking the Michaelis-Menten equation. The parameters of the equation can be readily interpreted as effectiveness$_{maximum}$ = 0.42, and dissociation constant = 0.17. It is usually very laborious to obtain these parameters from traditional regression modeling of the quantal effect histograms and cumulative histograms requiring data samples of at least 100 or so to be meaningful. The underneath figure shows an Excel graph of the fitted non-linear function for the data, using Newton's method (the best fit curve is here a hyperbola). A cubic spline goes smoothly through every point, and does this by ensuring that the first and second derivatives of the segments match those that are adjacent.

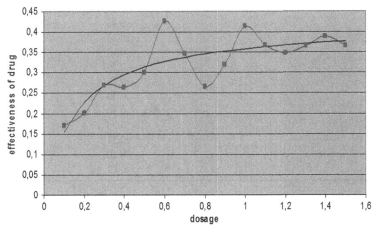

The Newton's equation better fits the data than traditional modeling with linear, logistic, quadratic, and polynomial modeling does as shown underneath.

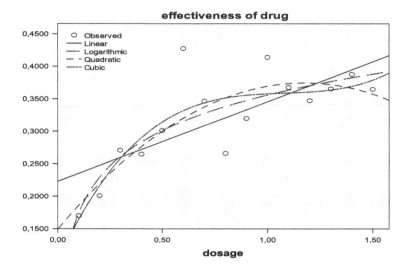

20.3.2 *Time-Concentration Study*

Time	Quinidine concentration µg/ml
0.10	0.41
0.20	0.38
0.30	0.36
0.40	0.34
0.50	0.36
0.60	0.23
0.70	0.28
0.80	0.26
0.90	0.17
1.00	0.30
1.10	0.30
1.20	0.26
1.30	0.27
1.40	0.20
1.50	0.17

The above table gives the data of a time-concentration study. Again a non-linear regression using Newton's algorithm is performed. We use the online Nonlinear Regression Calculator of Xuru's website. We copy or paste the data of the above table into the spreadsheet, then click "allow comma as decimal separator" and click "calculate". Alternatively the SPSS file available at extras.springer.com entitled "chap20newtonmethod" can be opened if SPSS is installed in your computer and the copy and paste commands are similarly given. For the data given 10 statistically significantly ($P < 0.05$) fitting non-linear functions were found and shown. For further assessment of the data an exponential function, which is among the first 5 shown by the software, is chosen, because relevant pharmacokinetic parameters can be conveniently calculated from it:

$$y = 0.41 \, e^{-0.48x}.$$

This function's measure of uncertainty (residual sums of squares) value is 0.027, with a p-value of 0.003. The following pharmacokinetic parameters are derived:

$0.41 = C_0 =$ (administration dosage drug)/(distribution volume)
$-0.48 =$ elimination constant.

Below an Excel graph of the exponential function fitted to the data is given. Also, a cubic spline curve going smoothly through every point and to be considered as a perfect fit curve is again given. It can be observed from the figure that the exponential function curve matches the cubic spline curve well.

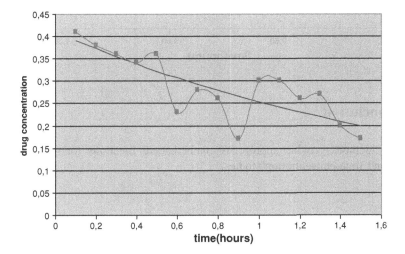

The Newton's equation fits the data approximately equally well as do traditional best fit models with linear, logistic, quadratic, and polynomial modeling shown underneath. However, traditional models do not allow for the computation of pharmacokinetic parameters.

drug concentration

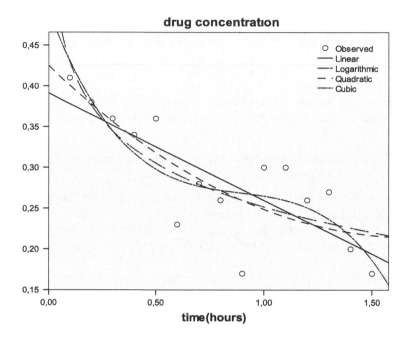

20.4 Conclusion

Newton's methods provide appropriate mathematical functions for dose-effectiveness and time-concentration studies.

20.5 Note

More background theoretical and mathematical information of Newton's methods are in Machine Learning in Medicine Part Three, Chap. 16, Newton's methods, pp 161–172, Springer Heidelberg Germany, 2013, from the same authors.

Index